Henrik Vejlgaard

LOOK THE AGE YOU FEEL

A MAN'S GUIDE TO LOOKING YOUNGER

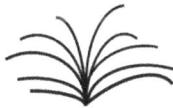

CONFETTI PUBLISHING

Look the Age You Feel

2nd edition, 2017

Book interior designed by Anette Damsgaard Bonde

ISBN-10: 1-939235-36-7
ISBN-13: 978-1-939235-36-7

Library of Congress Control Number: 2013914654

Published by Confetti Publishing

www.confettipublishing.com

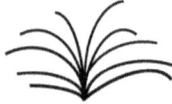

IMPORTANT NOTICE/DISCLAIMER
The contents of this book are intended to be entertaining in the tradition of magazine articles and are NOT intended and should NOT be relied upon as recommending or promoting a specific method, diagnosis, or treatment by physicians or other health professionals. The publisher and author specifically disclaim any liability, loss or risk, personal or otherwise, which is incurred as a consequence, directly or indirectly, of the use and application of any of the contents of this book.

CONTENTS

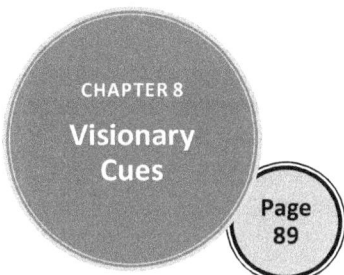

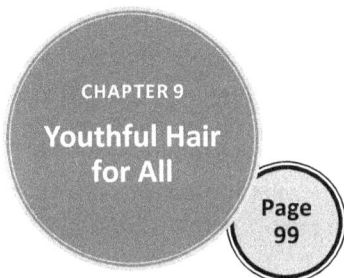

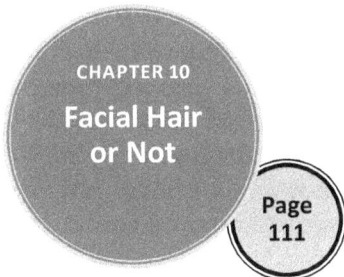

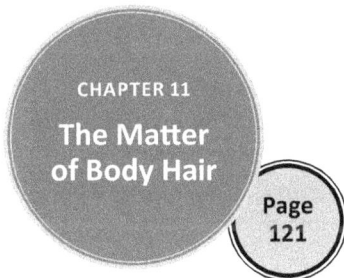

Understanding How to Look Younger

You are not the only one who wants to look younger. Millions of men feel the same way. All have very good reasons for this: They *feel* younger than they look. Now you have the chance to look the age *you* feel. With this book, you will get inspiration and guidance on all the options that are available to you if you want to look younger.

There are many ways to start looking younger. Some of these options you may be aware of, but with this book, you will not only get a complete overview of all options but also inspiration and guidance on how to make the best of them.

When we want to look younger, we have to be aware of the many signals or clues that give away our age. In particular, what we wear gives away our age. This book is about using these signals and clues to give a youthful impression to the world. Many will be surprised by how much younger they can look by just changing a few of these signals and clues.

The book is not about getting to look a certain age. It is a book that recognizes that people are different and have different needs and different attitudes towards their age. In order to help you in the best way possible, you must start by taking the Self-Perceived Age Quiz in the next chapter. The quiz helps you establish your desired visual age.

TOOLS AND GUIDELINES

When you know your desired visual age, you can start using the tools and guidelines in the book. The tools and guidelines have been created to help you no matter your biological age. But if your biological age is between forty and seventy years, you will probably stand to benefit the most from this book.

The Self-Perceived Age Quiz and the other tests and tools in this book are unique and have been developed by the author of this book. You will not have encountered the tests and tools in other books or magazines.

When you use it, you will realize that the book is like having your own personal style consultant at your disposal. But this style consultant not only guides you on how to look good, but more importantly, also how to look *younger*. We can look good at any age, but looking younger takes a whole different approach than just looking good. It takes an in-depth knowledge of the mechanisms that determine what youthfulness is.

SURGERY NOT REQUIRED

Cosmetic surgery is often thought of as one of the most effective ways of looking younger. Whether you have had cosmetic surgery or not—or will in the future—you will be able to benefit from this book. However, the focus of the book is to guide and inspire you in what you yourself can do to look the age you feel, both what can be done actively to look younger and what can be done to prevent some of the signs of aging. The book does *not* give advice on cosmetic surgery, but there are brief overviews of some medical and dental options available to people who want to look younger.

Look the Age You Feel is full of easy-to-use instructions. Please be aware that the book is focused on looking younger. It is *not* a book about the basics of general skincare, grooming, or health. Therefore, you will *not* find advice on, for instance, general hair care, or how to shave.

You can read the entire book, or you can just pick and choose the information that you feel you need most right now; at other times, you may want to read other parts. The content is structured so that if you are looking for specific information, it is easy to get an overview of each chapter right from the start of the chapter.

What Kind of Research Is the Book Based on?

The tests, tools, and guides in this book are based on the research and thinking of three books, all by the author of *Look the Age You Feel*. These are *Anatomy of a Trend*, which is about trends and trendsetters; *The Lifestyle Puzzle*, which is about the signals that our clothes and accessories tell other people about us; and *Style Eruptions*, which is about how changes in style take place. All three books are based on meticulous observation of thousands of women and men of different ages.

Specifically, this book is based on three different kinds of research:

❖ Studies of what constitutes what is young and youthful in our society.

❖ An understanding of how style changes and insight into trends that affect many people.

❖ Research on all the different things you can do to look younger.

CHAPTER 1

Finding Your True Age

CHAPTER FOCUS
* ❖ Biological age
* ❖ Self-perceived age
* ❖ Desired visual age

You know how old you are according to your birth certificate, but how *young* do you feel? Before you can start using the information and tools in this book, take some time to determine what age you want to convey to other people. This may be somewhere between your biological age and the age you feel you are. By thinking not only of our biological age but also our self-perceived age, we can meaningfully start working on our visual age—the age we want to convey to the people we meet. Now it is time to find the age you want to look!

Age is no longer just about our biological age, as determined by the date on our birth certificate. Today many people feel that they are younger than the age that their birth certificate says they are. For some, it is just a few years; for others, it can be several decades. No matter how many years, it is only natural that we want to *look* the age we feel.

Feeling young, dressing young, and acting young is not limited to a certain age. There are no rules anymore that say you can only do certain things at a certain age. No matter what your age is, as long as you are fit, you can go roller-skating, scuba-diving, and travel around the world.

We all feel and see that our bodies and faces change as we grow older. Sixty percent of general aging is due to genetics, which we can do little—or nothing—about. The remaining forty percent depends on how we live our lives. For example, work, stress, worries, sun bathing, and smoking influence how we look. This also means that we have some influence on a rather big part of the aging process.

We are not as limited by our biological age as we were in past centuries. These days, many people have jobs that do not require hard physical labor. This means that wear and tear on the body is different for many people as compared to fifty years ago. The result is that we often do not look or feel our biological age.

Age Elasticity

We have introduced the term *age elasticity* for the phenomenon in which you see yourself as younger than your biological age. Age elasticity is the difference between

❖ Biological age: the age according to your birth certificate.

❖ Self-perceived age: the age at which you perceive yourself.

Today, a person's self-perceived age is most likely younger than his or her biological age. A person's biological age may be forty-five years, but his self-perceived age could be thirty-five—or even younger.

You do not have to have a certain age elasticity to use the information in this book, but the higher your age elasticity, the more you can probably gain from the book's tools.

Age elasticity applies to both women and men. But, generally, men's age elasticity is higher than women's. It is not uncommon for men in their fifties to see themselves as being twenty-five years old. There are different reasons for men's higher age elasticity; the main reason probably is that men can father children for more years than women can give birth to children (at least the natural way).

HOW WE FEEL ABOUT AGE

For both sexes, it can be disturbing to look in the mirror and see an "old" person when you feel so young inside. This, of course, we want to correct so that we look the age we feel. Men's high age elasticity also makes us sensitive to how our wives and girlfriends look. If a husband and wife are both fifty years old, but the husband feels like a twenty-five-year-old and sees a fifty-year-old woman when he looks at his wife, he may feel there is an imbalance. Though he may himself look like a fifty-year-old, he may be attracted to someone who is closer to his self-perceived age. This explains why, after a divorce, a man may end up with a woman who is younger than his first wife is and younger than himself. (For some women, this is just an extra good reason to get to look the age they feel.)

Find Your Self-perceived Age

If your biological age is between thirty and seventy years, you can take the Self-Perceived Age Quiz to get an indicator of your perceived age. The test will reveal if your perceived age is younger or older than your biological age.

Self-Perceived Age Quiz

Your Biological Age (state your age)	__ Years
If you mostly associate with people who are younger than you, deduct	- 2
If you think you look younger than your biological age, deduct	- 3
If you mostly associate with people who are older than you, add	+ 3
If you truly enjoy experiencing change in your life, deduct	- 3
If you have two or more friends who are more than 10 years younger than you, deduct	- 2
If you live in a city with more than one million inhabitants, deduct	- 1
If you consider yourself conservative in most respects, add	+ 3
If you are curious about what is new in design and style, deduct	- 3
If you buy new, fashionable clothes at least every six months, deduct	-4
If you embrace most new technological developments, deduct	- 2
If you enjoy vacationing in big cities, deduct	- 1
If you are open-minded about how teenagers live their lives, deduct	- 3
If you have not changed your style of dress in the past 10 years, add	+ 3
If you have the same opinions that you did when you were in your 20s, add	+ 2
If you think that everything was much better "in the good old days," add	+ 5
Your approximate self-perceived age	

You know your biological age, and now that you also have an indication of your self-perceived age, you can use this to calculate the age that you want to convey to the world, that is, what you want your visual age to be. The first step in establishing your desired visual age is calculating your suggested visual age. This can be done using the Visual Age Calculator.

Visual Age Calculator

To find your suggested visual age, add your biological age to your self-perceived age and divide by two.

You can choose to convey your self-perceived age or suggested visual age, but if you have a very high age elasticity, you may feel more comfortable with choosing your desired visual age, which is your own modification of your suggested visual age.

EXAMPLE 1

Peter
- ❖ Biological age: 50
- ❖ Self-perceived age: 30
- ❖ Suggested visual age: 40
- ❖ Desired visual age: 40

EXAMPLE 2

Mark
- ❖ Biological age: 61
- ❖ Self-perceived age: 39
- ❖ Suggested visual age: 50
- ❖ Desired visual age: 40

When determining your self-perceived age, you can use the Self-Perceived Age Quiz as inspiration, but you may have a strong feeling yourself of what your self-perceived age is, and this is the number you should use as your self-perceived age in the calculation:

My biological age: _____

My self-perceived age: _____

Suggested visual age: _____

My desired visual age: _____

TALKING ABOUT YOUR AGE

Now that you have a precise idea what age you would like to look, you can start working on your visual age. This is what the rest of this book will help you to do.

But before you start changing your look and style, you should also be aware of how you talk about your age.

If you don't want people to know your biological age and want them to think that you are younger than you are, it does not make sense to tell them your biological age. You should consider avoiding talking about your biological age unless absolutely forced to.

This is not about *not* celebrating your birthdays, and it is not about lying. But when asked about your age, it is perfectly all right to indicate your self-perceived age, not your biological age. If people do not ask for specifics, then *you* choose what age you want to talk about. If you look more like your self-perceived age than your biological age, it actually makes more sense to talk about your self-perceived age.

If asked directly about your age, you can say, "I can tell you my self-perceived age…" or "Age is not in the skin but in the mind—and my mind is only xx years old" or "I have stopped talking about my age because age is such a relative concept."

Sometimes, we inadvertently reveal our age by stating the number of years we have been doing this or living there, such as, "I have lived in this apartment for thirty years." If you are around sixty years old, you can give the same information by saying, "I have lived half my life in this apartment." In this way, you can avoid talking about numbers.

Not all people may be aware of the different concepts of age—but more and more people are becoming aware of age elasticity because they feel it themselves.

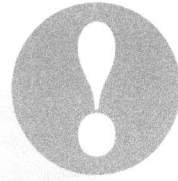

On your way to looking younger

❖ Acknowledge your self-perceived age.

❖ Choose a visual age between your biological age and your self-perceived age to look convincingly youthful.

❖ Avoid talking about your biological age.

CHAPTER 2

How Not to Reveal Your Age

CHAPTER FOCUS
- ❖ Guessing a person's age
- ❖ Different approaches to looking younger
- ❖ Options overview

When you have determined your desired visual age, you want to start changing other people's perceptions of your age. First, you have to know the signals that reveal your age. Then you have to learn how to take advantage of them. It's about using visual signifiers to signal our desired age, but also about reversing and disguising your biological age and sometimes even preventing the changes. There are many options in dealing with age-revealing signals. Luckily, we are in complete control of most of them.

Many men who live in the public eye know the importance of looking younger, and some are very good at looking (much) younger than their biological age. They can be actors, singers, or television personalities. Often we know the biological age of these men (which can make it difficult to be objective about guessing their age), but most people would say that they look younger than their biological age.

Like these men, you can also learn to look younger no matter your biological age. And you will have one advantage over them: People that you meet in public will not know your actual biological age, so it will be easier for you to convey your desired visual age.

The first step in changing people's perceptions of your age is to understand exactly what it is that reveals our age. Both our face and our body are affected by biological changes as we grow older. For most people, these changes first become visible in the face. Often the changes in the body are felt and become visible to others a decade or two later than those affecting the face. The slower visual aging process of the body is a great opportunity for us. It means that we can draw attention to the body—and away from the face—without drawing attention to yet another age revealer. We can use the body to help us signal that we are younger than we are.

We also have to be aware of the many style signals that can reveal our age and sometimes reveal much more than our body. For different reasons, many people do not pay as much attention to the style signals as they do to the body's signals, and consequently, they may end up missing some options that can take years off their age.

We have psychology to help us understand the possibilities the body gives us when we want to look younger. Experts in body language have studied how we look at other human beings when we meet them. Whether we are meeting people for the first time or meeting someone we know well, we use the "vertical scanning approach." When you meet someone, you normally do not just look in the person's eyes. You also look at the person's face and body. Both women and men use the vertical scanning approach, but women use it much more conspicuously than men do.

The Vertical Scanning Approach

When we meet someone, and we want to have a closer look at that person—for whatever reason—we typically start by looking in their eyes. Then we divert our eyes to the upper torso, and then back to the eyes.

Then we divert our eyes again, and this time we may look at the person's hands before looking back to the eyes or face.

Then we look at the hair and then the eyes again.

When we are observing someone or talking to someone for a longer time, we will take in more and more of the body.

Many people also look at the feet of another person and look at the shoes he or she is wearing.

There are many different reasons why we use the vertical scanning approach. Some people are shy or don't want to be thought of as flirting. Many people are also naturally curious about what the person is wearing. So they observe. In some cases, their look will be admiring; in other cases, it's the opposite. There are undoubtedly many other reasons why we don't just look at the face of the person we are talking to or of a stranger we are meeting for the first time. But in all instances, we use the vertical scanning approach.

This non-verbal interaction is so very common that we hardly think about it. But it reveals how important what we wear can be to other people's perceptions of us; we can use this to control our image.

The vertical scanning approach is a great opportunity in the quest to look younger because, in this way, we can cue people as to our age using many different clues, not just the skin of our face. Especially from a distance, the body plays a bigger role, not only because it is larger than our face, but also because what we wear is full of clues that other people decode and use to start forming an opinion before we are face to face.

AGE PERCEPTIONS

Imagine you see a woman in the distance. She appears to be forty years old. You guess her age based on the way she dresses, her hairstyle, and the way she moves. From psychology, we know that first impressions count—and that it is in the human mind to want our first impressions, consciously or unconsciously, confirmed. As the woman gets closer, you will automatically want to confirm that she is a forty-year-old woman.

If, in fact, her biological age is fifty, you may think, "Well, for a forty-year-old, she looks her age." You may also adjust your thinking and say to yourself, "Maybe she is forty-five years old." The point is that the way she dresses and the way she moves have made her look younger in your mind, and will probably have done the same in many other people's minds.

On the other hand, if the woman approaching you is only thirty years old, you will think, "Why does she dress older than she is?" or perhaps, "Wow, she looks fantastic for someone who is forty." Again, the message is that our clothes, our hairstyle, make-up, and other visual signals hold strong clues for other people about our age.

This is something that we men also can take advantage of when we want to convey how old—or rather, how young—we want to look. The first step is about being aware of the different types of age-revealers and learning how to approach them. You can see different types of age-revealers in the Age-specific Age-revealers Chart.

Age-specific Age-revealers Chart

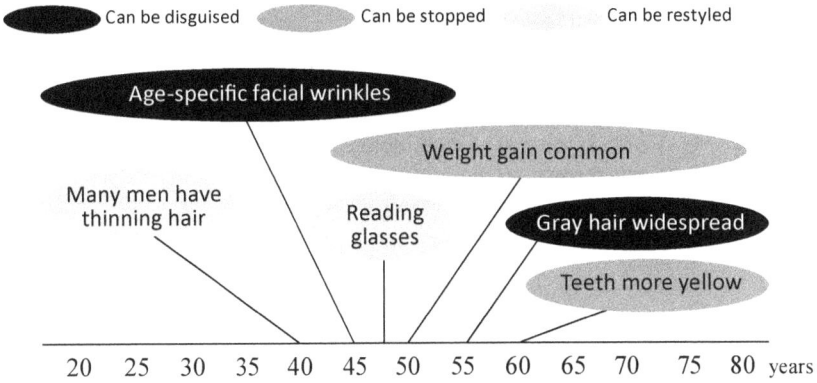

Can be disguised   **Can be stopped**   Can be restyled

Age-specific facial wrinkles

Weight gain common

Many men have
thinning hair

Reading
glasses

Gray hair widespread

Teeth more yellow

20   25   30   35   40   45   50   55   60   65   70   75   80 years

Options Overview

Theme	Chapter
Accessories	6
Arms	3
Body	3
Body hair	11
Clothes	5
Eyes	8
Facial hair	10
Hair	9
Lifestyle	13
Mentality	14
Posture	3
Teeth	7
Weight	3

4 Different Approaches to Looking Younger

There are different approaches to looking younger that you will learn about in this book:

❖ You can prevent (some) biological changes.
❖ You can reverse the biological changes.
❖ You can disguise the biological changes.
❖ You can use visual signifiers to look youthful.

Prevent the biological changes
Preventing biological changes in our body is not easy, but having healthy eating habits and doing sensible exercise on a regular basis can get us a long way.

Reverse the biological changes
Knowing what causes aging gives us a chance—in some cases—to do something about visual aging. We *can* prevent some of the aging of our skin and of our body. For instance, weight gain can be stopped or reversed. We can also do something about the yellowing of teeth.

Disguise the biological changes
Wrinkles and gray hair are two very typical biological age revealers that can be disguised. For instance, in the case of gray hair, this can easily be disguised by coloring the hair. In the case of age-specific face wrinkles, they, too, can be disguised (e.g., with correctly sized *and* trendy eyewear frames).

Use visual signifiers to look youthful
We use visual signifiers to convey our age and deflect attention from the biological changes. Clothing, hairstyles, eyewear, and facial hair are typical visual signifiers, but there are many others that you will be introduced to in this book. For instance, we do not have to use reading glasses when we need eyesight correction. There are other options. And for hair length, we can decide the length of our hair ourselves.

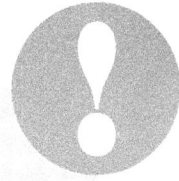

On your way to looking younger

❖ Be sure to get an overview of all your options and then choose what will work for you.

❖ Be aware of the age revealers that you yourself can do something about.

❖ Use the visual signifiers that will make you look younger.

3

Looking at the Body

CHAPTER FOCUS
❖ Weight
❖ Height
❖ Posture
❖ Skin

When they want to look younger, many people focus on the face and underestimate what the body reveals about their age. But just as most people know what a young face looks like, they also know what a young body looks like. In everyday life, we notice that young people are slimmer and have better posture than old people do. In other words, the body is one big giveaway of our age— with or without clothes. In this chapter, we will look at the body without clothes, so to speak. And in the following three chapters, we will look at the body with clothes.

We learn to interpret certain signs about the body from personal experience, from watching people, and from what we learn from medical science and through the media. Therefore, when we look at a person's body, there are several signs that reveal to us the person's age.

Again and again, we can observe that people put on weight as they grow older. Statistics confirm this, and science explains that one reason for this is that our metabolism changes as we grow older. Therefore, most of us are aware that young people—in general—tend to be slimmer than older people.

Statistics also document that each new generation born since World War II has been taller than the previous one. Today, the average young man is taller than his father and grandfather. Therefore, many people are aware that young men tend to be taller than older men.

Sports and exercise are something that we mostly see young people do, and we notice that there are fewer old people doing sports and exercise. This also helps confirm that young men tend to have fitter bodies than older men.

BODY LANGUAGE

As we grow old, our body language changes. We become more hesitant, we have less flexible bodies, and we are less agile.

The good news is that we men can prevent this from happening or at the very least we can reverse some of the changes. It may not be easy, but it can be done—with exercise. We know that exercise is good for us for many reasons—our health, our wellbeing, and so on. But we should not forget our body language because our body language has a huge influence on one of the most important aspects of our lives—our sexuality.

With our body language, we send signals of sexual agility and virility. We become aware of this when we look in a full-body mirror. We should be aware of our own body language. It is certainly noticed by other people.

SIGNS OF AGING

The skin on our faces changes, and so does the skin on our bodies. With age, the skin on the body becomes wrinkled, and liver spots develop, may also show up on many parts of the body. Again, we are well aware that younger men tend to have smoother skin than older men do.

So, we know what makes us look older in the eyes of the world (and in our own eyes as well). On the other hand, we also know what can make us look younger:

❖ If you are slim, you are younger looking.
❖ If you are tall, you are younger looking .
❖ If you are fit, you are younger looking.
❖ If you are agile, you are younger looking.
❖ If you have a good posture, you are younger looking.
❖ If you have all your hair, you are younger looking.
❖ If you have smooth skin, you are younger looking.

The first step in changing people's perceptions of our age is considering these facts. If something can be done on one or more of these aspects of the body, it can help you look younger.

Let us take a closer look at each element and see what can be prevented, what can be reversed, and what can be disguised. There are, inevitably, things that you cannot do anything about. Don't be frustrated by this because there are so many other things that you can do something about.

WEIGHT ISSUES

Most people gain weight as they grow older, often because our metabolism changes. If we keep eating the same number of calories as we grow older that we ate when we were young, we will eventually gain weight. There are also other reasons people gain weight, and there are many good reasons to avoid it. Health is one of them, but it is also about looking youthful.

Weight Control Program

If you want to prevent weight gain, avoid gaining *more* weight, or lose weight you have gained as an adult, you should adopt the Weight Control Program. This program is not about a certain diet. It is about changing habits.

Shopping habits

❖ Buy food that is high in protein. One gram of protein contains only four calories per gram. One gram of carbohydrates also contains four calories. Though proteins and carbohydrates contain the same number of calories it is better to get more protein than carbohydrates for two reasons. 1) You will stay fuller for a longer period of time when eating protein. 2) Calories from carbohydrates may come from sugar and other fast carbohydrates, of which we do not need a lot. Too much sugar is stored as fat. One gram of fat contains nine calories, and one gram of alcohol contains seven calories. If you eat 100 grams of protein and feel full, you have consumed only 400 calories. If you eat 100 grams of fat and then feel full, you will have consumed 900 calories. In both cases you feel full, but you will have gained less weight by eating proteins than fats.

❖ In general, avoid buying packaged food that does not have a nutrition facts label. With a nutrition facts label, you can learn how much fat, carbohydrates, or protein you will be eating.

❖ In general, avoid buying food that contains a lot of fat. On average, a maximum of 30% of the number of calories in the food you buy should come from fat.

❖ Be critical when buying "light" or "diet" products. Some light or diet products contain lots of sugar. If you eat more sugar than your body can use, you will gain weight.

Eating habits

❖ Avoid fatty and oily foods whenever possible; that is, when you have an option to choose something else, do so.

❖ Avoid butter, margarine, mayonnaise, and similar fatty foods whenever you can; that is, when the food has not already been prepared.

❖ Avoid sugar as much as possible. That is, avoid soft drinks, candy, and other sugary drinks and food. If you want to snack, eat fruit or vegetables instead.

- ❖ Eat fibers often, and especially in the morning. This will keep you full longer.
- ❖ Avoid fast food, not only because it is generally more fattening than regular food but also because we eat fast food quickly with the risk of overeating.
- ❖ Avoid low-calorie soft drinks. They can trick your body and brain into feeling hungry. Drink water and/or skim milk instead. Sometimes you can drink fruit or vegetable juices as an alternative.
- ❖ If you use food to comfort yourself, prepare food with as few calories as possible.
- ❖ Don't avoid foods that you really like even if the food is "bad" for you. However, try to eat it at special occasions, for instance, when you are celebrating.
- ❖ Even if you eat healthy food, you should never eat any more food than what it takes to make you feel full. Even healthy food contains calories that will make you gain weight.
- ❖ Avoid snacking between breakfast and lunch. Often, snacking between breakfast and lunch is more about habits than about being hungry.
- ❖ It is better to eat several small meals than a few big meals—as long as you don't take in more calories when you eat those small meals. In this way, you will not get to feel so hungry that you eat more than you need.

Mealtime habits

- ❖ Eat slowly—actually eat as slowly as possible. It takes about 20 minutes for your brain to register that your stomach is full. When your brain has registered that you have food in your stomach, the hunger will go away.
- ❖ Stop eating before you feel full. If your stomach is full after 10 minutes of eating, it will be about 20 minutes before your brain will tell you to stop eating. This means that you can go on eating food that you don't really need. The slower you eat, the less risk of overeating.
- ❖ Only eat when you are hungry, but try to avoid waiting to eat till you are very hungry because you are then more likely to eat more before your brain registers that you are full.
- ❖ Never bring all the food to the table, whether you're eating out of pans or off of plates. When not socializing, leave some food in the kitchen.

- ❖ Separate food from entertainment. We eat faster when we watch television because we don't talk, and because we eat faster we will end up eating more than we need.
- ❖ Avoid using big plates for dinner. It will make you put more food on the plate. Use small ones instead.
- ❖ Eat with a small fork and/or small spoon. This will make you eat more slowly.
- ❖ Be conscious about taking a second helping—don't make it a routine to have seconds.
- ❖ Eat meals that consist of a maximum of two courses when not socializing.
- ❖ In every twenty-four-hour period, make sure that there are at least eight hours during which you do not eat. For most people, this means not eating during the night.

CHANGE YOUR HABITS PERMANENTLY

If you need to make major adjustments in your diet in order to stop gaining weight or to lose weight, change one or two habits at a time. To change all your habits at once can be hard. For many people, it will be more effective in the long run to stop one weight-gaining habit every two weeks or every month. Shopping habits should be changed right away.

If you follow the basic anti-weight gaining information above, it does not matter what specific kind of diet you choose, if any. The important thing is that you eat and drink fewer calories than you burn.

If you want to be successful in achieving your weight goals, it is important to change your habits permanently, not just temporarily. But be sure to change them in a way you can sustain for a long time. If you are really unhappy with what you eat, there is a greater risk of getting back to habits that will make you gain weight.

HEIGHT

The statistics speak loud and clear: Young men of today are taller than the previous generation. Sometimes you can see three generations of men next to each other, and the youngest man will almost always be the tallest. So we learn to associate being tall with being young.

The thing about our height is that once we are fully grown, there is not much we can do about it. However, we know that if you are tall, you are younger looking. Therefore, there is nothing wrong for a man to want to add some height to his height if that is what he wants in order to look younger. Here are some suggestions for men who want to add some extra height:

Be aware of the height of heels on your shoes

The heels on men's shoes can vary, either because of the type of shoe or because of fashion. A casual loafer will often have a very low heel or no heel, whereas a more formal loafer will have a regular heel. If you want to have as much height as possible on your heels (without making a big deal out of it), just be aware of the differences in the height of heels of shoes that you would normally use.

Add an extra outsole

Some men have an extra outsole added to their brand-new shoes because they want to make them as robust as possible so they last longer (typically the outsole gets worn down before the rest of the shoes). This process can add a quarter of an inch to the heel of a shoe. So if you would like a little extra height to your heels, just make your shoes more robust with an extra outsole.

Use regular insoles

If a shoe does not fit because it is a little too big, an insole is the way to deal with making the shoe more comfortable. It will also add a little height, not much in itself, but if combined with the other options you will be able to feel the difference. If you plan on using insoles on a regular basis, you may want to buy shoes that are a half size bigger than your normal size.

Use height-adding insoles

We all have different walking styles, and in some cases our foot may need some extra support one way or another. Some people often need a so-called support insole that is made especially for them in order to avoid injuries when walking or running. Some support insoles will be about getting an insole that is high at the end of the sole. If you would like to add a little height to your height, you can get a support insole with extra height, even if you do not need a support insole for health reasons (though that can be your excuse when asked).

Make cowboy boots part of your style

Cowboy boots are one of the few boot styles for men that are born with extra heel height. The design of the heel of the cowboy boot came about because a high heel would make the boot stay put in the stirrups when galloping over the prairie. In other words, the height of the heel of the cowboy boot is not about vanity; it is about functionality.

Cowboy boots are an iconic American style. They may be in or out of fashion but they will always be around. One interesting thing is that cowboy boots come in many different styles and colors, and there are cowboy boots that will match blue jeans and cowboy boots that will match a tuxedo and everything in between. Some men simply like the cowboy boot style so much that they choose to wear them almost all the time, both with casual and formal clothes. Most likely it is not about getting the extra height. But if a man would like to have some extra height, he can just make cowboy boots his style and wear them as much as he likes, and disregard the fact that they may not always be in fashion. (And if asked why he wears them, he can say he likes the style.)

There are so many other options for men to look younger that most men will just ignore the height issue, but for men who want to add some extra height, the above options are viable because many men who do not care about their height actually avail themselves of these options. Therefore, these options will not be cause for any embarrassment.

THE FIT BODY

Depending on where you live and where you go on vacation, you will probably be wearing clothing that will show some skin—maybe a t-shirt or a polo shirt. This is when you also reveal how fit your body is and something about your biological age. There is no doubt that a fit body is younger-looking than a non-fit body.

If you want to change the looseness of your skin and the contours of your body, exercise is an important activity. There are many ways to stay fit, and it does not matter what kind of exercise you choose, as long as it achieves what you want to achieve and you are motivated to do it regularly. It is better to do a little exercise that you really like than something that you will try to skip. If you want to work on the looseness of your skin and the contours of your body, you can get inspiration from the Fit Body Activity Guide.

The Fit Body Activity Guide

Activity		Firmer Skin	Muscle Definition
	Weight control program	X	
	Walking/race walking	X	Lower body
	Jogging	X	Lower body
	Bicycling	X	Lower body
	Aerobic exercise	X	X
	Stair-climbing machine	X	Lower body
	Swimming	X	X
	Rowing (also in machine)	X	X
	Training with weights or machines	X	X

Worth Knowing: Liposuction

If you want to have a fit-looking body and don't have the time or patience to go through weight control and/or exercise, liposuction may be an alternative. Liposuction is the removal of fat cells by surgery. Liposuction is mostly used to remove fat deposits from the hips, stomach, and thighs, but can be done in many areas of the body and the chin. The surgical procedure removes the fat and reduces the number of fat cells in the area so that fat will not come back so easily in this area. Liposuction should be performed by an experienced plastic surgeon.

There are many reasons to focus on doing exercises—sports and exercise can be fun, your health improves, and you get a young-looking body. There are also many reasons why people do not keep fit: lack of time, lack of energy, and lack of knowledge are some of them.

If your aim is to have a fit body in order to look younger—and you have reasons for not doing any kind of full-body exercise—you can get away with less: just focus on the arms. While focusing on the arms will not improve your overall health, it can help you look younger. The arms are important because they are the part of the body that is most likely to be visible to other people when you wear a T-shirt or a polo shirt.

The upper arms are the big age revealer of the upper body. The upper arm consists of two muscles: biceps and triceps. If these two muscles are firm, this can help signal a youthful, firm body.

It is never too late to start working on the muscles of the upper arm. At almost any age, they can get firmer. So if you cannot do any other kind of exercise, the Basic Biceps and Triceps Exercise Program will help you have firm upper arms. The exercises can be done almost anywhere at any time.

Basic Biceps and Triceps Exercise Program

The exercises should be done every second day when starting the program. After three months, the program can be continued two to three times a week, depending on how toned you want the arms be. Warm up by swinging your arms back and forth twenty-five times, both to the sides and up in the air.

Biceps Exercise
Arm bending with dumbbells
1. Sit down on a chair without armrests with your legs wider apart than the shoulders.
2. Place your left hand on your upper left leg for support.
3. Place the right elbow on the upper right leg for support.
4. Let your right arm hang down with the dumbbell in your right hand.
5. Raise your right arm to your chest while getting elbow support from the upper leg.
6. Lower the right arm to starting position.

Do ten repetitions with right arm, then ten repetitions with the left arm. Do this three times in all.

Triceps Exercise
Push-ups on knees
1. Lay down on the floor on your stomach.
2. Lift your feet off the floor, but keep your knees on the floor.
3. Cross your ankles.
4. Place your hands on the floor underneath your shoulders.
5. Raise your arms so that you lift your upper body.
6. Keep the body straight while lowering the arms.
7. Be careful not to lock your elbows when arms are stretched.

Do one set of eight to ten repetitions.

It is best to use dumbbells when doing the exercises.
If you have not done any biceps or triceps training before,
you should probably only start with six-pound dumbbells and
then use heavier weights as you get stronger. Always
stop exercising if you feel any kind of discomfort.

The more physical exercise you do,
the better, of course. If you have limited
time, focus on the upper body.

BEING MORE FLEXIBLE

When we grow older, our body language also changes. We move more slowly and our movements become more hesitant. Generally, this has to do with the body becoming less flexible. When this happens, we often become more careful with physical activities. While being careful is always wise, it is also wise to work on keeping the body as agile as possible. Being flexible will make you feel better and look younger.

The good news is that inflexibility can be reversed. In one study on how to improve flexibility, two groups of men were compared to each other. One group was comprised of teenagers and the other of seniors (aged 63 to 88). The study documented that both groups could become more flexible with equal ease.

The best way to stay flexible and agile is doing sports and exercise. If that is not an option, the Dynamic Movement Exercise Program is a good alternative. Dynamic movement consists of many different exercises that will make you stay flexible and improve coordination.

Dynamic Movement Exercise Program

The exercises should be done twice a week. Warm up by hopping up and down twenty-five times.

Rolling Down

1. Stand upright with feet placed wider than the shoulders.
2. Raise your arms out to the sides, a little higher than horizontal position.
3. Relax your knees.
4. Slowly bend your head and arms towards the floor.
5. Slowly continue rolling your head towards the floor, letting the arms move to the floor first.
6. Try to let the fingers touch the floor (bend the knees if necessary).
7. Roll slowly up to starting position.

Repeat exercise three times.

Sitting Cross Reach

1. Sit down on the floor with your back straight, legs straight in front of you.
2. Place your left arm behind your back as support, legs straight in front of you.
3. Raise your right arm and slowly move it towards your left foot.
4. Bring back right arm and use it as support behind your back.
5. Raise your left arm and slowly move it towards your right foot.

Repeat ten times.

Standing Diagonal Reach

1. Stand up with feet apart.
2. Bend the right leg while the left leg is stretched out to the side.
3. Place the right hand on the right knee.
4. Place the left hand in front of the lower right leg.
5. Slowly bring the left arm across your chest and up in the air.
6. Bring left arm back to starting position.

Repeat five times with left arm, then change position and do the exercise five times with the right arm (left leg bent, right leg stretched).

GOOD POSTURE

Flexibility plays an important part in good posture. People with good posture signal alertness and youthfulness—no matter their biological age.

Slumping and a drooping head are two signs of old age. Both can happen for many different reasons, though biology and bad habits are the major culprits.

If bad posture is about bad habits when working or relaxing, there is only one way of improving the posture: change the habits and be conscious of standing, sitting, and walking as erectly as possible. The Dynamic Movement Exercise Program will also help improve posture.

In some cases, a "shoulder strap" can be used to stand more erect. A shoulder strap will press the shoulders back to their natural position. If bad posture is a serious problem, a specialist should be consulted.

On your way to looking younger

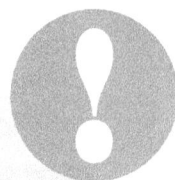

❖ Staying slim has many benefits—looking younger is just one of them.

❖ Muscular upper arms are important in signaling a youthful body.

❖ Beware of succumbing to bad posture.

CHAPTER

4

Test Your Fashion Profile

CHAPTER FOCUS
- ❖ Style study
- ❖ Fashion attitudes
- ❖ Test yourself

The most important step on your way to looking younger is wearing the right clothes. Clothes are one of the body's big age revealers–but the great thing is, we can control this age revealer ourselves. By constantly adapting our style to what is trendy, we have countless opportunities to convey our desired visual age. But first you have to find out if your current style is sending the signals that you want to convey.

Whether we care or not, just by wearing clothes, we send signals to the rest of the world about our age. Clothing is not just about function–clothes have become very important in our communication with other people. This lifestyle aspect has become more important because we do not all wear the same type of clothing. There are many different styles, and each style sends different signals to the people around us. The one signal that matters to people who want to look younger is what the style reveals about their age.

In order to find out what your style reveals about your age, you have to identify your style preferences. This is done by taking the Style Preference Test. The test will reveal if your style is doing the job you want it to—to look younger—or if you need to make adjustments in order to wear clothes that make you look younger. The test is about the colors, patterns, fabrics, and types of clothing items that you prefer and that are normally part of your wardrobe or that represent your preferred style.

Style Preference Test

The test consists of ninety different style-related terms and descriptions arranged in ten sections. Choose one term/description in each section that best describes your style. Any particular choice does not mean that you have to wear the style, just that you like it. If you don't think that there is a term/description that fits your style, choose what comes close or skip the section.

1. Colors

  a. O Beige
  b. O Blue
  c. O Pastels
  d. O Purple
  e. O Bright colors
  f. O Brown colors
  g. O Faded colors
  h. O Do not care
  i. O What's in fashion

2. Patterns

a. ○ Do not like patterns
b. ○ Very discrete patterns
c. ○ Floral patterns
d. ○ Paisley
e. ○ Leopard patterns
f. ○ Native American patterns
g. ○ Tie-dye
h. ○ No preference
i. ○ What's in fashion

3. Fabrics

a. ○ Linen
b. ○ Tweed
c. ○ Knits
d. ○ Velvet
e. ○ Shiny fabrics
f. ○ Leather
g. ○ Sweatshirt fabric
h. ○ What's practical
i. ○ What's in fashion

4. Clothing Items

a. ○ Turtleneck
b. ○ Trench coat
c. ○ Quilted jacket
d. ○ Scarves indoors
e. ○ Fur coat
f. ○ Leather pants
g. ○ Cargo pants
h. ○ Sweat clothes
i. ○ What's in fashion

5. Decoration on Clothes

a. ○ Do not like decoration on clothes
b. ○ Monograms
c. ○ Patterns of diamonds in diagonal checkerboard arrangement
d. ○ Embroidery
e. ○ Rhinestones
f. ○ Fringes
g. ○ Frayed
h. ○ What's functional
i. ○ What's in fashion

6. Accessories

a. ○ None
b. ○ Tie
c. ○ Straw hat
d. ○ Beret
e. ○ Gold jewelry
f. ○ Cowboy hat
g. ○ Bandana
h. ○ Baseball cap
i. ○ What's in fashion

7. Shoes

a. ○ Penny loafers
b. ○ Wingtip shoes
c. ○ Tassled shoes
d. ○ Blunt-toed shoes
e. ○ White loafers
f. ○ Cowboy boots
g. ○ Sneakers
h. ○ Comfortable shoes
i. ○ What's in fashion

8. Jewelry

a. ○ Don't wear jewelry
b. ○ Signet ring
c. ○ Gold bracelet
d. ○ Necklace with oversize pendant
e. ○ Gold and diamonds
f. ○ Leather
g. ○ Organic materials
h. ○ Mix of different jewelry
i. ○ What's in fashion

9. Silhouette

a. ○ Fitted clothes
b. ○ Tailored suits
c. ○ Trousers with pleats
d. ○ Loose-fitting clothes
e. ○ Tight clothes
f. ○ Close-fitting clothes
g. ○ Baggy clothes
h. ○ Without suit jackets
i. ○ What's in fashion

10. Style Preference

a. ○ Understated
b. ○ Classic
c. ○ Old-fashioned
d. ○ Sculptural
e. ○ Glamorous
f. ○ Outdoorsy
g. ○ Hand-made look
h. ○ Casual
i. ○ What's in fashion

Count the number of times you have crossed off each letter (a to i) and place the numbers in the score box.

Score Box

Letters	Number of times crossed off
a	
b	
c	
d	
e	
f	
g	
h	
i	

In the Style Preference Test Key, you can learn what your style preference is. The key divides style into two categories: static styles and dynamic styles. The styles that are static rarely change, and the styles that are dynamic change often according to trends and fashion. Generally, dynamic styles will make us look younger. Some static styles are currently neutral to age, and some will make the wearer look older.

Often people dress in a mix of static and dynamic styles. Or some may prefer one style at one time and another style at other times. But, generally, many people prefer to dress in a style that is similar or somewhat similar to one of the nine styles presented in the Style Preference Test.

When we want to look younger by using the way we dress, we have to focus on the dynamic styles. These are the styles that hold the most youthful signals simply because they represent styles that are changing. If you want to look young, you have to change your way of dressing from time to time because whenever there is a new generation of young people, they create new styles of dress–and their styles have the strongest youthful signals.

Style Preference Test Key

If you have an equal distribution of choices, you can either go through the test again and be more critical of your answers or choose the key answer that you feel best resembles your actual style.

- Only or mostly a's: Your style preference is for sporty clothing and/or a minimalist style in clothing. This is a static style, but this style is mostly neutral to age.

- Only or mostly b's: Your style preference is classic. This style is static and is not optimal if you want to look younger. You should adjust your style to a more dynamic style that will help you look younger.

- Only or mostly c's: Your style preference is romantic. This style is static and is not optimal if you want to look younger. You should adjust your style to a more dynamic style that will help you look younger.

- Only or mostly d's: Your style preference is bohemian. This style is static and is not optimal if you want to look younger. You should adjust your style to a more dynamic style that will help you look younger.

- Only or mostly e's: Your style preference is glamorous. This is a static style but this style is mostly neutral to age, unless it is hip hop glamorous, which is youthful.

- Only or mostly f's: Your style preference is what can best be described as rugged or outdoorsy. This is a static style, but this style is mostly neutral to age.

- Only or mostly g's: Your style preference is what can best be described as organic and/or street style. This is a static style, but this style is mostly neutral to age.

- Only or mostly h's: Your style preference is very casual or practical/functional. This style is static and is not optimal if you want to look younger. You should adjust your style to a more dynamic style that will help you look younger.

- Only or mostly i's: Your style preference is trendy. This means that the style is very dynamic and signals a youthful style.

Today, it makes a lot sense to dress in a style that matches the age that we feel. If you are fifty years old but feel forty, this should be reflected in the way you dress. But how does a forty-year-old man dress? Or, for that matter, how does a man in his twenties, his thirties, his fifties, or his sixties dress? It is obvious that even though some men are the same age, they do not necessarily dress in the same way; however, there are some typical ways of dressing for each age.

In the next chapter, you will be guided on how to find the current season's style that is right for you, based on your desired visual age.

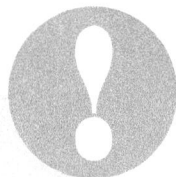

On your way to looking younger

❖ Pay a lot of attention to your style.

❖ Use clothes to make yourself look younger.

❖ Accept that your style has to change from time to time.

CHAPTER 5

Dress Your Desired Visual Age

CHAPTER FOCUS
❖ Focus on trends
❖ Age-specific styles

Understanding the principles and influence of trends means that we have the knowledge to dress in a way that many people consider fashionable, stylish, and youthful. By associating ourselves with current fashion trends, we can send some very youthful signals about ourselves. By following the guidelines in this chapter, you can easily get the style that matches your desired visual age.

More and more people are becoming aware of fashion trends— the changes in style and taste that we see at certain intervals. Many fashionable trends are first adapted by young people, and when this happens, they are worth paying attention to because clothing and all the other style elements that are under the influence of trends hold strong signals about our age.

If we want to look younger, we can use knowledge of trends from the books *Anatomy of a Trend* and *Style Eruptions* to change other people's perceptions of our age.

The new styles that end up affecting many people are first adopted by the trendsetters (who are the people who first start wearing something new). Many trendsetters are in their twenties and thirties, but also people in their forties, fifties, and sixties can be—and are— trendsetters. But the trendsetters who are in their forties, fifties, and sixties are often copying the trendsetters who are in their twenties and thirties. By doing so, they get to look much younger than other men in their forties, fifties, and sixties who do not follow what is fashionable.

Changes in fashion happen regularly. However, it is not always easy to figure out exactly which style signals what age.

In fashion, there are two phenomena that influence how we dress: fads and trends. When a new style appears, one of two things can happen: the style will be popular for one season and then disappear. Then it was just a fad. Or it can go on being popular for several years, and then it becomes a trend. There is a big difference between fads and trends, and this we can take advantage of when we want our clothing to reflect our desired visual age.

If we are talking about high fashion from the famous fashion brands in Europe and in North America, their style changes so fast that only a few people register that there was a new style. When this is the case, there is really no point in using their styles to signal your age because very few people will recognize them and know how to interpret them. So if we want to use clothes and accessories to our advantage in looking younger, we have to avoid the fads that will be out of fashion in a few months' time (at the time when these designers introduce a whole new style).

Though many fashion fads are adopted by young people—and could be used to signal youthfulness—they are not really reliable because six months later they will be out of style, and the rest of the world will not know what this or that style represents in terms of youthfulness. In that way, trends are much more reliable because many people will be aware of the trendy styles and know that this style represents what is new (which equals what is young).

Trends have a longer time span and, therefore, we can also better document them—and count on them to help us signal the age that we want to signal.

Trendy styles will be popular for a long time. They will not be popular with the same people all the time, but the popularity of the trendy style will flow from the trendsetters to the rest of the population during a period of time that can be anything from three to ten years.

Fashion changes, and any style photos in this book would be outdated within a couple of seasons. Therefore, you will not find any fashion photos in *Look the Age You Feel*. To get updated on what is fashionable, read one or two fashion magazines for men, either printed versions or the online versions. Choose the well-known magazines to be sure to get news on what is trendy now.When looking for inspiration, look at the fashion magazines' fashion editorials because they will show clothing and accessories that are in stores (when the magazine was published). Fashion show photos, that is, photos from the presentation of the clothes to fashion buyers and the fashon media will not necessarily show clothing items that are in stores and much of the clothing that is presented during the fashion shows will not go on to become a trend. Therefore, fashion show photos are not nearly as relevant as the fashion magazines editorials.

While there are many online fashion resources, you cannot be sure that they are right for you: the photos may be outdated or be more representative of a style in another part of the world than where you live. No matter where you live, you can generally trust US, British, and French men's magazines to represent men's global fashion trends.

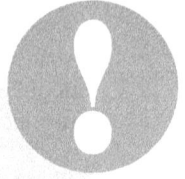

On your way to looking younger

❖ Go for a style that matches your visual age.

❖ Avoid going for a look much younger than your self-perceived age.

❖ Be aware that you have to update your clothing style on a regular basis to radiate youthfulness.

CHAPTER 6

Flaunting Your Youthful Image

CHAPTER FOCUS

❖ Accessories overview
❖ Shoes
❖ Watches

Accessories are powerful visual signifiers. Even though accessories are only a part of what we are wearing, they play a much bigger part than their actual size. Accessories are popular and there are a lot more trendy and fashionable accessories to choose from than ever before. The accessories have to look good with what you are wearing but they also have to make you look the visual age you want to convey. With the right accessories, you can further flaunt your youthful image.

Clothes and accessories play an equally important part in signaling our age to others. Clothes are the basic tool you can use in communicating your visual age, and accessories can be used to refine this communication. With our clothes, we can give a very good indication of our age but often it is the accessories that underline peoples' perceptions of our age.

There are many different types of accessories. Basically, the types of accessories that are available to us are these:

❖ Hats
❖ Sunglasses
❖ Glasses
❖ Earrings/studs
❖ Bags
❖ Necklaces
❖ Watches
❖ Bracelets
❖ Rings
❖ Belts
❖ Shoes

All accessories are not equally important, either in our wardrobe or in being age signifiers. Sometimes it is better *not* to wear certain types of accessories because they may make you look older. Here is a short overview of what the different accessories can do for you when you want to look younger.

Hats

Hats are worn for functional and decorative reasons. Out in the sun, however, it is important to wear a hat or cap if you want to protect yourself from the sun's rays. Of course, out in the cold it is also important to wear a hat. On special occasions, such as weddings and funerals, hats are sometimes worn. Hats can also be part of what is fashionable, and then certain styles of hats will be popular.

Sunglasses

Sunglasses are important not only for protecting the area around the eyes from the sun's wrinkle-advancing rays but also because they are important in signaling your desired visual age.

Glasses

Some people need glasses to see; other people can use eyewear as a way of looking younger—if they wear the right type of eyewear. More on this in Chapter Eight.

Earrings/studs

In the past it symbolized a rebellious attitude in a man if he had an earring. This has changed today because earrings/studs are much more of a fashion statement. If earrings/studs are in fashion, they can be used to signal youthfulness just as any other accessory. Whether they are used by men or women, earrings and studs are powerful visual signifiers because they are close to the face. If you do not want extra attention to your face, do not wear earrings/studs.

Rings

Most people who are married wear a wedding ring. This you should wear no matter the style or what it says about your age. The important signal here is that you are married! But for all other rings, be aware that they are fashion accessories that are under the influence of trends. Not just the style but also the number of rings is under the influence of trends.

Necklaces

Some men who wear necklaces do this for very personal reasons. Sometimes the necklace has a religious pendant. Normally a necklace is covered by clothing and it does not really matter what kind of necklace, if any, a man wears. It has rarely been the case, but sometimes necklaces become fashionable. If you are comfortable wearing a necklace, do as the young men do.

Watches

Watches are practical and essential to many people, not only because they tell the time but also because they can be used to underline one's style. A watch is, of course, an accessory, and to some, a piece of jewelry. But watches are also an important conveyer of age.

Bracelets

Most men do not wear bracelets but sometimes bracelets for men become fashionable. And many young men will then be wearing a bracelet. If you are comfortable wearing a bracelet, do as the young men do. If not, there are other ways to imitate them.

Bags

Bags have become a very important accessory that can be used to convey your desired visual age. Go to the online StyleGuide to find out about the bags that are trendy this season.

Belts

In some cases, belts are part of what is fashionable, and then they should be used like other fashionable accessories.

Socks

Most men prefer dark-colored socks. Some choose a sock in a color that matches the color of the shoe. Some choose a sock in a contrasting color. Since socks are not very visible, it is not something that you need to pay a lot of attention to. Dark-colored socks will rarely send the wrong signals.

Shoes

Shoes are perhaps the most important accessory we have at our disposal if we want to look younger. As we grow older, there is a tendency towards wearing more comfortable shoes. If comfortable shoes convey youthfulness, then this is perfect, but that is rarely the case. Go to the online StyleGuide to find out about the shoes that are trendy this season.

FACE PIERCINGS

Face jewelry includes eyebrow piercings and nose piercings. Piercings became popular in the 1990s, and because face piercings were first adopted by young people (including many teenagers), they do hold strong signals about youth. Actually, face piercings are such strong signals for teenagers that they will not work well for someone over the biological age of forty. Face piercings are the exception to the rule that you should try to wear what young people are wearing if you want to look younger than your biological age. Also, face piercings may draw attention to wrinkles in the face that you don't want attention drawn to (if you want to convey another age than your biological age).

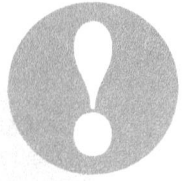

On your way to looking younger

❖ Pay a lot of attention to accessories (because people observing you do).

❖ Be aware that all or most of the accessories

must come from the same age group to look convincing.

❖ Avoid face piercings, as they can draw attention to parts of the face where you do not want

Facing Your Face

CHAPTER FOCUS
❖ Skin
❖ Teeth

From a distance, the body is the big revealer of age, but close up, the face becomes the major age revealer. There are several things that can be done to convey a youthful face. No matter your age, the most important thing you can do is to stop the biological age revealers from progressing. Second, there are more and more options that can help reduce wrinkles. Because teeth age much like the skin unless well taken care of, there is also guidance on how to get the most youthful smile.

With age, the skin on the face becomes thinner, drier, and more fragile. This affects the texture of the skin. One of the first signs of this change is also the most revealing sign of aging–wrinkles. Even though not all wrinkles are due to signs of aging–unless we consider smiling a lot a sign of aging–a youthful appearance of the face becomes the number one priority for many people who want to look younger.

It can be shocking to look in a mirror and see the reflection of our biological age and not our self-perceived age. Sometimes we ourselves are bothered the most by this difference–and that is a very good reason to do something about it.

To some people, cosmetic surgery is the solution to bring balance between biological age and self-perceived age. While plastic surgery can bring some remarkable changes to the face, maybe even making it more or less wrinkle-free, it is also important to be aware that wrinkle-free is not necessarily the same as young or youthful. If a person continues to use clothing and make-up that is typical of his biological age, he will not look a lot younger, just wrinkle-free.

As more and more people also know the telltale signs of men who have had facelifts, we can end up in a situation in which the facelift becomes, in a way, an age revealer in itself. People will think to themselves: "I can see he has had a facelift, so probably he is actually twenty years older than he looks." Therefore, a facelift gives the best results when used along with youthful visual age signifiers. Of course, these age signifiers are also very powerful *without* plastic surgery.

Telltale Signs of a Facelift
❖ An unusually high forehead
❖ Eyebrows unusually high on the forehead
❖ Stretched skin between eyelids and eyebrows

Wrinkles

What most people notice about aging skin are the wrinkles. There are two different kinds of wrinkles:

❖ Dynamic wrinkles: wrinkles that appear in the face when talking, smiling, grimacing, etc.
❖ Static wrinkles: wrinkles that are visible even when not moving the face

Dynamic wrinkles are wrinkles that people of almost any age have. When we smile, we get wrinkles around the eyes, or we may make a grimace that will make a wrinkle in the forehead appear.

Because faces, skin structures, skin colors, and our lives are all different, the types of wrinkles that are dynamic and those that are static will vary from face to face. Many of the wrinkles around the eyes start out being dynamic. As age progresses, there will be more and more dynamic wrinkles, and the wrinkles that used to be dynamic will become static. There are several reasons for this. One reason it that with 22 muscles around the eye and 10,000 blinks per day, this part of the skin is in constant movement. Another reason is that the outer layer of skin around the eyes is extremely thin. It measures just one fourth of the thickness of the skin on the rest of the face. The consequence is that it dries out twice as quickly as the rest of the face.

The type of wrinkles that bother people varies from person to person. But if we take a general view, there are two sub-categories of wrinkles:

❖ **Primary Age-Revealing Wrinkles**
  "Crow's feet"
  Drooping eyebrows
  Drooping eyelids
  Pouchy eyes
  Mouth wrinkles

❖ **Secondary Age-Revealing Wrinkles**
  Forehead lines
  "Worry lines"
  Nose-to-mouth wrinkles

Typical Face Wrinkles

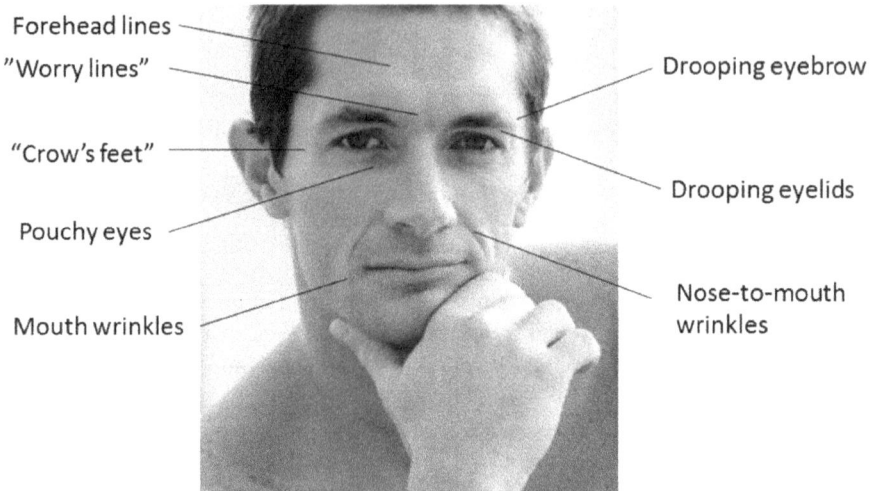

Forehead lines
"Worry lines"
"Crow's feet"
Pouchy eyes
Mouth wrinkles

Drooping eyebrow
Drooping eyelids
Nose-to-mouth wrinkles

It is often the wrinkles around the eyes that bother people the most because this area often represents the first visual change in the skin.

Today we know a lot about how and why the skin ages. A part is due to biological processes that we can do very little to reverse. But how we live our lives also affects our skin, and this we can do something about.

The skin's firmness relies on two very important connective tissue fibers, collagen and elastin. These fibers are interwoven and very elastic. They make it possible for the skin to snap back again—in the same way an elastic band will snap back—when stretched. If we want to avoid losing these tissue fibers, we have to look at what destroys the skin's collagen and elastin. Some of the collagen and elastin is destroyed in natural biological processes. But a major part of the collagen and elastin is destroyed by

❖ Sunlight
❖ Tobacco smoke
❖ Pollution
❖ Stress

Sunlight is responsible for most of the skin's aging. Dermatologists believe that the UV rays present in ordinary daylight are responsible for more than 2/3 of the skin's aging.

You can compare the aging of the skin to leaving an elastic band outside in the sun for too long. After a while, it will lose its elasticity. Exactly the same thing happens with our skin when exposed to the sun. The more exposure to the sun, the quicker the loss of elasticity in the skin.

HOW TO AVOID GETTING WRINKLES

If you want to reduce the number of lifestyle-induced wrinkles, you should do the following:

Moisturize with Sunscreen

The sun does a lot of good to sustain life on earth. So humans, animals, crops, etc., need the sun. The sun also provides vitamin D to humans, one of the vital vitamins that we do not always get enough of through food. Therefore, we cannot and should not avoid the sun altogether. However, there is no doubt that the sun causes wrinkles. Therefore, we should get as little direct sunlight as possible on the face. This is ensured by using a moisturizer containing sunscreen.

Sunscreens have different Sun Protection Factors (SPF). SPF is a numerical sunscreen rating system that is used all over the world. SPF numbers on products in stores go from 4 to more than 100. More on which SPF to use later in this chapter.

No Sun Tanning

Being tanned is not particularly youthful since people of all ages like to tan. And tanning will cause wrinkles. When you tan, this is also a sign that the sun has affected your skin in a way that also causes wrinkles. Therefore, if you want to avoid wrinkles, the basic thing is not to tan. This does not mean that you cannot stay out in the sun. You just have to protect your skin from the sun with sunglasses, a hat with a brim, and sunscreen with the highest possible SPF. The best sunblock is non-transparent clothing. The next best is a sunscreen cream, gel, or oil. Most sunscreens should be applied 20 minutes before you go outside so that it has time to work. If you sweat a lot, the sunscreen has to be reapplied often—how often will depend on the type of product (cream, gel, or oil) and the SPF number. The lower the number, the more often the sunscreen has to be reapplied.

Avoid Direct Sunlight

The sun is damaging to the skin no matter where you are. Of course, when the sun is shining, it is not always easy to avoid direct sunlight. But staying directly out in the sun should be avoided as much as possible. If you stay out in the sun, you should, as mentioned, wear sunglasses and a sun hat or cap with a brim, and use a sunscreen with Sun Protection Factor.

The face is the part of the body that is exposed to the sun the most. However, the sun affects the skin on the body in the same way as the skin on the face. But as most people have their body covered with clothing during much of their lives, there are typically fewer sun-induced wrinkles on the body. People who sunbathe a lot or work outside unclothed without sunscreen can also get wrinkled skin on the body. Sunscreens should be used on all parts that are exposed to the sun.

When choosing a sunscreen, it is important to make sure that it filters both types of ultra-violet rays. There are two types of rays that reach the earth: UV-A and UV-B.

❖ UV-A rays penetrate deep into the skin and will destroy the skin's collagen and elastin and cause wrinkles.

❖ UV-B rays are stronger than UV-A rays; they cause redness in the skin and cause skin cancer.

Both types of UV-rays will cause you to tan, but UV-B will make the skin go red. Therefore, many sunscreens only protect against UV-B in order to avoid your skin getting red while allowing UV-A rays to pass so that the skin can tan. Suncreen that only protects against UV-B will make your skin wrinkle.

Sunscreens with para aminobenzoic acid or cinnamates protect against UV-B rays. A sun cream, gel, or oil must contain zinc oxide, titanium dioxide, avobenzone, or benzoefurans in order to protect against UV-A rays. Also benzylidene camphor to some degree protects against UV-A rays.

If you are concerned about wrinkles and skin cancer, a sunscreen cream, gel, or oil should protect from both types of UV-rays. The information label should clearly state what kind of protection the sunscreen offers, either by stating that it contains a UV-A filter, a UV-B filter, or both. If it does not, you should find a sunscreen that clearly states what types of rays are filtered.

Darker skin types do not get sunburned as easily as lighter skin types do, but the UV-A light ages the skin in just the same way. Therefore, everybody—regardless of their skin color—should use sunscreen if they want to reduce the risk of wrinkles. In the Skin Type/Sunscreen Guidelines on the next page, you can see which SPF you should use if you do not want to get wrinkles from the sun. The guidelines clearly show that no matter what skin type you have, you should use SPF with double-digit numbers. Sunscreen rubbed on the skin will typically work for at least a couple of hours and must be reapplied according to the label instructions.

Skin Type/Sunscreen Guidelines

If preventing wrinkles is your priority, you should use a sunscreen with both a UV-A filter and UV-B filter.

Skin Type	Description	Recommended SPF
1	Very light skin, reddish hair	Minimum 80
2	Light skin, blond hair	Minimum 80
3	Olive-colored skin, brown hair	Minimum 50
4	Brown skin, dark brown hair	Minimum 50
5	Dark brown skin, black hair	Minimum 30
6	Black skin, black hair	Minimum 30

Tanning Beds

Tanning beds or similar artificial tanning devices work in the same way as the sun, and they cause wrinkles just as the sun does. How many wrinkles depends upon the tubes in the tanning bed. The tubes can transmit both UV-A and UV-B rays, or just UV-A rays or just UV-B rays. The rays have different effects on the body, as mentioned earlier. UV-A rays are the cause of wrinkles and UV-B rays are the cause of skin cancer. The kind of rays transmitted in the tanning bed is up to the owner of the device who puts the tubes in. The lettering on the tubes should reveal what kind of rays they transmit. If there is no clear indication what type of rays a tube transmits, the device should not be used under any circumstances. If you do not want to get wrinkles, you should not use tanning beds or other tanning devices.

Smoking

Tobacco smoke causes wrinkles. The tobacco contains substances that destroy the collagen and elastin of the skin.

Cigarette smoke speeds up the aging of the skin, especially at the corners of the eyes and around the mouth. Heavy smokers typically are five times more wrinkled than non-smokers who do not breathe in smoke.

If you want to reduce the number of lifestyle-induced wrinkles, you should not smoke. If you smoke, you should stop smoking. It is never too late to benefit from stopping smoking. There are several types of stop smoking aids available at drug stores if you want to stop smoking.

We know more and more about passive smoking and the perils that passive smoking contains. Passive smoking can cause cancer, cardiovascular diseases, and many other ills—as well as wrinkles. Depending upon how long you are in a smoke-filled environment and how much smoke there is, the smoke will get inside your body and do damage. If you want to reduce the number of lifestyle-induced wrinkles, you should avoid all passive smoking.

Pollution

Pollution—from exhaust fumes to factory smoke—can alter the skin because it changes how the cells in the skin divide and renew themselves. Pollution can, in fact, accelerate the production of cells that cause the ageing of the skin through a series of chemical reactions, which can end up causing wrinkles. Daily cleansing of the face with a mild soap before bedtime and using a moisturizing gel or cream in the morning are the basics of skin protection, whether you live in a polluted area or not. More than one facial or body wash with soap in 24 hours will remove the grease that the skin creates naturally as a protective barrier against pollution. If—for general hygienic reasons only—you feel the need to wash your face and/or body more than once a day, use cold water only and for as short a time as possible, and moisturize often.

Stress

Being busy and having an active life does not influence the emergence of wrinkles in any extraordinary way. But serious stress can affect the skin and also end up causing wrinkles. Stress is a physical and emotional state that is highly negative to a person's health. It can lead to depression and anxiety, which may also end up causing wrinkles. Thus, there are many good reasons to deal with stress as early as possible.

Grimacing

Smiling, chewing, and squinting can also cause wrinkles. When we use our face to express ourselves—such as smiling and grimacing—we use the elasticity of the skin. Some wrinkles are unavoidable when using our face. Smiling is important and is, in many peoples' opinion, much more appealing than an un-smiling face. But some people have habits of wrinkling their forehead or the area between their eyes and other face muscles. The more they use these face muscles, the bigger the risk of the wrinkles there becoming permanent.

If you make faces a lot and you want to avoid the wrinkles this can cause, you have to train yourself to express yourself in other ways. But first you have to become aware of what extent you make faces. You can study yourself whenever you have the chance, look at photographs of yourself, and ask people that know you if they have noticed that you make faces more than the average person.

WHAT TO DO ABOUT WRINKLES

If you have wrinkles, there are several ways of making them less visible. What you want to do will depend upon how many wrinkles you have and where you have them. If you have age-related face wrinkles, you have the following options:

- ❖ Moisturizing
- ❖ Anti-wrinkle creams
- ❖ Botox
- ❖ Fillers
- ❖ Peels and scrapings
- ❖ Cosmetic surgery

These options work in different ways and can be used for different kinds of wrinkles. The methods can be combined. You can use the Age-Specific Anti-Wrinkle Treatment Guide to find out which biological age is *generally* relevant to the different treatments.

Age-Specific Anti-Wrinkle Treatment Guide

Biological Age / Treatment	20s	30s	40s	50s	60s	70s
Moisturizing	X	X	X	X	X	X
Anti-wrinkle creams		X	X	X	X	X
Botox			X	X	X	X
Fillers			X	X	X	X
Peels and scrapings				X	X	X
Cosmetic surgery				X	X	X

Moisturizing

How we treat our skin on the outside has very little to do with getting wrinkles. Deep wrinkles are caused by the sun, tobacco, pollution, stress, and by our genes. All this causes the skin to lose its elasticity. But when we moisturize the skin, we can temporarily erase or prevent the small and very delicate wrinkles caused by dry skin from being visible. Any cream can do this, but as soon as the cream wears off or is washed off, the wrinkles will again be visible. A moisturizer is effective for less than 24 hours.

If you have small and delicate wrinkles in the face, use a moisturizer that you like, without perfume. Gels have become popular moisturizers because they do not leave the skin shiny. You should use a moisturizer that contains a sunscreen if you are often outside.

Anti-Wrinkle Creams

Most anti-wrinkle creams work in the same way as moisturizers. They will only temporarily erase the small and delicate facial wrinkles from being visible.

Anti-wrinkle creams cannot erase wrinkles permanently simply because the molecules that are supposed to erase the wrinkles cannot penetrate the skin deeply enough to affect the skin. So even if the cream contains ingredients that should work on the wrinkles, the molecules in these ingredients cannot penetrate the skin, and, consequently, cannot erase any wrinkles. The skin has a phenomenal ability to prevent outside particles from penetrating it, therefore there is no cream that can *permanently* alter the structure of the skin and erase wrinkles. Anti-wrinkle creams only affect the small and delicate wrinkles, just like a moisturizer; in fact, most anti-wrinkle creams *are* just moisturizers.

Skin-Repair Treatments Overview

Type	Description	What it Does	How it Works	Results	Side Effects
Vitamin-A acid	Cream or gel with vitamin A, which was originally used as a very effective anti-acne treatment.	Smoothes fine facial wrinkles and blotches from sun damage. It will not affect dynamic wrinkles.	Changes the cellular metabolism of the skin's surface.	Only as long as it is used.	Red, itchy, and scaling skin. Sunscreen protection essential.
Glycolic acids ("fruity acids")	Cream or facial wash with natural fruit substances.	Smoothes rough, sun-damaged skin and fades age spots.	Sloughs away dried, sun-damaged skin on the surface.	Only as long as it is used.	Red and itchy skin. Sunscreen protection essential.

There are different over-the-counter products that contain Vitamin-A acid and glycolic acids, and they are marketed under different brand names.

Botox

Botox is one of several brand names for injections that contain botulinum toxin, a poisonous substance that, when injected in certain parts of the face, can smooth wrinkles. Generally both static and dynamic wrinkles can be treated with botulinum toxin; for instance, the worry wrinkles in the forehead, between the eyebrows, and around the eyes can temporarily be smoothed by botulinum toxin.

The doses for cosmetic use are very small and are not considered dangerous. However, this does not mean that there are no risks involved. Botulinum toxin will paralyze part of the face and, if injected wrongly, it can paralyze a wrong part of the face and can cause, for instance, a drooping eyelid.

Botulinum toxin injections only take a few minutes. Normally, it takes a couple of weeks to see the full effect of the injection. Depending upon how much botulinum toxin is used, the face will lose some of its natural flexibility. The effect will last three to six months and then the treatment can be repeated.

Fillers

Fillers are injectable collagen, hyaluronic acid, or fat that can fill deep, static wrinkles, typically between the eyes, from the nose to the mouth, and on the upper lip. The filler is injected into the wrinkle where it will fill out the wrinkle.

Fillers Overview

Type	Description	Results
Injectable collagen	Collagen derived from animal or human sources	Visible right away; lasts 2-6 months
Fat	Fat from patient's own body	Visible right away; lasts up to 6 months
Hyaluronic acid	Natural component in all living organisms	Visible right away; lasts up to 1 year

The fillers are sold under different brand names. There are other types of fillers than the ones mentioned in the Fillers Overview, but they are not as well established.

All fillers may have side effects, but they are generally rare and mostly mild. When the filler has been absorbed by the body, it has to be injected again to maintain the effect.

Peels and scrapings

Peels and scrapings remove "old" skin and let new skin grow. In both peels and scrapings, the outermost layer of the skin is affected, but by different means. You can get details of the differences in the Peels and Scrapings Comparison Overview.

Peels and Scrapings Comparison Overview

Type	Description	What It Does	Results
Chemical Peel	Surgical removal of the top layer of skin with a chemical solution. Different solutions are available.	Smoothes fine and/or coarse wrinkles, depending on chemical solution used.	Visible after skin has healed.
Dermabrasion (scraping)	Scraping away the outermost layer of skin with scraping device.	Smoothes fine wrinkles.	Visible after skin has healed.
Micro-dermabrasion (scraping)	Abrasion with a fine sandblaster on outermost layer of skin.	Smoothes fine wrinkles.	Visible after skin has healed.

Treatment is performed by a dermatologist or cosmetic surgeon and normally only takes a short time. But the healing process is slow. New skin has to grow and, at first, it will be pinkish. This can be covered with make-up until the skin gets a less pinkish skin tone. This process takes several months.

At-home peeling and scrapings kits are also available, but they have no effect on wrinkles. They will clean the skin and remove the dead skin cells, something that can also be done by a sponge rub. Excessive use can have side effects, including skin diseases such as rosacea and acne.

Cosmetic Surgery

Most cosmetic plastic surgery is not about getting a more youthful look—it's about adapting to society's and/or one's own beauty ideals.

This could be changing the shape of the nose or getting the ears tucked in. But the size of the nose or "big ears" has nothing to do with looking younger. The size of the nose is no clear indication of age. Young people have small noses and big noses. Older people have small noses and big noses. And the same goes for ears.

But cosmetic surgery also offers options in dealing with the signs of aging, in particular in the face. And these options can be a highly effective way of getting to look more youthful. The relevant procedures are presented in the Age-Reducing Facial Cosmetic Surgery Options Overview.

Age-Reducing Facial Cosmetic Surgery Options Overview

Surgical Procedure	Target Area	What It Can Do	What It Won't Do
Forehead Lift/ Brow Lift	Forehead	Smoothes out wrinkles in forehead; lifts eyebrows and eyelids; smoothes out furrows between eyebrows.	In some cases, upper eyelids may still be drooping after surgery.
Eyelid Surgery	Upper and lower eyelids	Removes excess skin or fat on upper eyelids and/or below the eyes ("bags").	It will not remove crow's feet or other wrinkles around the eyes, eliminate dark circles under the eyes, or correct sagging eyebrows.
Facelift	Cheeks, jowls, chin, and neck	Stretches the skin in the lower part of the face; removes sagging skin and smoothes out deep creases from between the nose and mouth; removes folds and fats around the skin and neck.	It will not remove excess skin or fat around the eyes.

You can go to the Age-Reducing Facial Cosmetic Surgery Options Pros and Cons to learn a few more details about the surgical procedures and some alternatives.

A person can have a wrinkle-free face through cosmetic surgery, but surgery cannot give a youthful style and attitude. A person may have fewer wrinkles, but if the person in question has not changed the other visual signals, people will not necessarily see a younger person. In other words, cosmetic surgery is no guarantee that other people will automatically guess that a person is any younger.

Age-Reducing Facial Cosmetic Surgery Options Pros and Cons

Surgical Procedure	Pros	Cons	Alternative(s)
Forehead Lift Eyebrow Lift	Can smooth out horizontal forehead wrinkles that cannot be smoothed out in any other way. Can affect two important areas at one time: horizontal wrinkles in forehead and drooping eyelids.	Risk of unhappiness with forehead area Risk of visible scars with short or thin hair Risk of infection.	Eyewear, learn more in Chapter Eight. Botox, learn more in this chapter Chemical peel, learn more in this chapter
Eyelid Lift	Can make eye area more youthful. There are not really any alternatives for drooping eyelids and heavy bags under the eyes.	Risk of unhappiness with eye area. Risk of visible scars with short or thin hair Risk of infection.	Eyewear, learn more in Chapter Eight
Facelift		Does not affect small and fine wrinkles around the eyes. Risk of unhappiness with eye area. Risk of visible scars with short or thin hair Risk of infection.	Botox, learn more in this chapter Fillers, learn more in this chapter Dermabrasion, learn more in this chapter Chemical peel, learn more in this chapter

SKIN DISCOLORATION

The color of the skin may also change as we age. Some of the color change may be "wear and tear," but there are also some changes in color that have other causes. In some cases, there are treatments available that will change the discoloration that sometimes comes with age.

Dark Circles

Dark circles under the eyes are often caused by very thin skin in the area under the eyes. The skin around the eyes is the thinnest on the face, and if a person has many visible blood vessels in this area, they can appear as purple circles under the eyes. In fact, it is blood that makes the skin dark. There are no treatments for thin skin and "dark circles" under the eyes.

If for any reason it is important that you disguise the dark circles under your eyes there are no other option than using a so-called concealer to cover the dark area of the skin. Pick one in your own skin tone.

An alternative to using a concealer is using eyewear to disguise the dark circles (read more on eyewear in the next chapter).

Bags under the eyes are often due to fat deposits and/or water. As the skin loses its elasticity, the bags can get "baggy." Plastic surgery is the only way to permanently get rid of bags under the eyes. In some cases, they can be hidden by using eyewear (more on this in the next chapter).

Red Spots

Rosacea is a skin disease that causes red spots in the skin, especially on the nose, the area around the nose, cheeks, and the chin. Without treatment, rosacea may get worse over time. Other skin diseases can also become more pronounced with age or start in adult life. An unusual amount of redness in the skin, especially on the nose, should be looked at by a dermatologist. In some cases, there are treatments available that will make the redness go away.

Pigment Changes

Pigment changes can happen because of sun damage to the skin or because of hormonal changes. Best known are hyper pigmentation or brown spots. Age or liver spots are a common form of hyper pigmentation that, for many people, are signs of aging. They are the result of damage by the sun. Hyper pigmentation can occur on the face, on the neck, on the hands, and all over the body.

Hyper pigmentation can be reduced by prescription creams that lighten the skin; most contain hydroquinone, which bleaches darkened skin patches so the dark spots gradually fade to match normal skin coloration. Prescription bleaches contain twice the amount of hydroquinone, the active ingredient, as over-the-counter skin bleaches. In severe cases, there are other creams with tretinoin and a cortisone cream that a doctor can prescribe.

Hyper pigmentation can, in many cases, also be removed by laser by a medical doctor. This will not scar the skin, but a test spot in an inconspicuous place will need to be done, as laser removal sometimes make spots worse instead of better.

Broken Blood Vessels

If a person is spending a lot of time outdoors, wind, sun, and other weather influences can cause broken blood vessels in the face, in particular on the nose and on the chin.

Today, broken blood vessels can be treated with a laser. When the destroyed blood vessels are treated with a laser, they go away. After one treatment, there will be a reduction in broken blood vessels. Depending on the number and type of broken blood vessels, more than one treatment may be needed.

COLOR OF TEETH

Most people equate white teeth with youth. This is only natural because with age, our teeth often do change color. They become more yellow or grayish. There are several reasons for this. Some families have yellower teeth than the average population, and this will progress with age. In most cases, however, it is due to wear and tear. What we eat and drink and how we take care of our teeth cause the teeth to change color.

How to Avoid Getting Yellow/Gray Teeth

If you want wear and tear to affect your teeth as little as possible, there are several things you can do:

No coffee, tea, cola beverages, or red wine
All drinks, hot or cold, that contain strong color will discolor teeth if consumed repeatedly. This is true for coffee, tea, soft drinks like brown-colored cola, and red wine. Milk or water, either bottled or tap, are the best alternatives to soft drinks.

No smoking
Smoking will also discolor teeth. The more a person smokes, the stronger the discoloration. Just look into a cigarette filter to see what kind of color tobacco from one cigarette can create. Cigarette smoke will often make teeth gray.

Brushing
Brushing your teeth once every 24 hours is considered the gold standard of dental care. It must be done before going to sleep after having used dental floss. Some people do not feel fresh before having brushed their teeth in the morning after breakfast. But this cannot substitute brushing your teeth before going to sleep. Then you just have to brush your teeth twice a day.

HOW TO GET WHITER TEETH

Brushing is, of course, the everyday procedure to keep teeth and gums healthy. For general dental care, the toothpaste should contain fluoride. There is no indication that "whitening tooth pastes" will make your teeth whiter. But there are several ways a dentist can help make your teeth whiter. These are the most popular ways:

Dental Cleaning

Regular dental appointments are good for many reasons. During regular dentist appointments, the dentist can clean the outside of the teeth with extra rough toothpaste and remove tartar that can cause discoloring. Done regularly, this will help keep teeth white, though this will not make teeth bright white.

Bleaching

There are different kinds of bleaching methods. The dentist can do the bleaching at the clinic, or the patient can get a do-it-yourself kit to use at home. When done at the clinic, the patient gets a whitening gel rubbed on the teeth (set for about one hour). During that time, the dentist will use a special lamp to put light on the teeth as part of the whitening process.

At-home treatment starts with the dentist making an imprint of the teeth that is turned into soft silicone "dentures" that can be filled with a whitening gel and put in the mouth, typically overnight. This is done every night for several weeks.

Veneers

Veneers made of porcelain can be used as a new facade on teeth. To some extent, veneers can be compared to getting new enamel on the front of the teeth in the color and shape that you want. Veneers are ultra thin and very strong. If placed on a tooth correctly, they will stay in place for many years.

Gums

Receding gums are also a sign of aging. Receding gums can be a result of disease, in which case there are treatments available. If a person has receding gums, it is in some cases possible to cover the teeth with gum again. The extent to which this is possible depends on the quality and health of the gums and teeth.

Tooth Fillings

One sign of aging that is often overlooked are teeth fillings and silver and/or gold teeth. Young people have had fewer dental procedures done to their teeth because it is with age that you get dental problems that result in fillings, etc. In the twentieth-century, silver fillings and silver or gold teeth were the materials used to deal with cavities and other dental disease. This has changed dramatically—today there are other alternatives that make it harder to detect fillings and artificial teeth in the mouth. Silver fillings and metal, artificial teeth can be replaced by tooth fillings made of plastic materials.

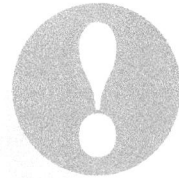

On your way to looking younger

❖ Be aware of what makes your face age and prevent this from happening or worsening.

❖ Study your face to find out what makes you look older.

❖ Take advantage of what you can control yourself.

Visionary Cues

CHAPTER FOCUS
❖ Contact lenses
❖ Laser surgery
❖ Eyewear

Carefully chosen eyewear can be used to make you look younger in different ways. The design of the frame can hide age-revealing facial features, but it can also send some very youthful signals—much more so than other accessories because this accessory is worn in a way that all people you meet will notice. In other words, eyewear can effectively be used to cue people you meet as to your desired visual age.

Until we are in our forties, it is only a minority of people who need to have their vision corrected. Among those who need their vision corrected, there seem to be two schools of thought: Either you appreciate the extra style opportunities that eyewear gives you or you wear contact lenses (or get surgery). There are several reasons why many people dislike eyewear. Some cannot find frames that look good on them, many associate eyewear with getting old, and for others there are practical considerations due to their job or leisure activities.

Luckily, there are alternatives if you do not want to wear eyewear to correct your vision. But if you choose to wear eyewear, it is worth knowing that when chosen carefully, eyewear can be used to make you look younger in different ways.

The circumstances for needing eyewear or other vision correction can come early in life. Then it is either about being farsighted (you cannot read and see things at a close range) or about being nearsighted (you cannot see things at a distance). In the Vision Correction Guidelines, you can get an overview of your options to correct your vision. Some people who are either farsighted or nearsighted also have some kind of misshaping of the eye's lens. This is called astigmatism, which can also be corrected.

With age, most people need reading glasses. Many people realize when they are in their mid-to-late forties that they have trouble reading. This is due to a biological and completely natural process. In young people, the lens in the eye is soft and flexible, and readily changes shape to focus. Over time, there is a gradual hardening of the tissue making up the lens. As a result, the lens's ability to focus decreases steadily. The medical term for the reduction in eyesight is called presbyopia, but it is also popular to refer to it as "old-age vision."

People in their forties sometimes believe they have become farsighted when they suddenly find that they cannot read anything in small print but can still read street signs and watch movies comfortably. The exact cause for farsightedness is not fully known, but we know that old-age vision is the result of the lens becoming less flexible. In the Vision Correction Guidelines, you can also see what your options are if you need to have your vision corrected because of presbyopia.

Vision Correction Guidelines

Correction Method	What Can Be Corrected	Pros	Cons
Contact Lenses	Farsightedness Nearsightedness Astigmatism Old-age vision	With contact lenses, no one can see that you use vision correction. You can get contact lenses that function as reading glasses.	You may not be able to wear contact lenses at all times.
Laser Surgery	Some mild cases of farsightedness Nearsightedness Astigmatism Old-age vision (in this case, specifically a technique called Monovision)	After surgery, you will have "normal" vision.	Surgery can go wrong, and there's a risk that you will have to wear glasses even after surgery.
Eyewear	Farsightedness Nearsightedness Astigmatism Old-age vision	You can use glasses to your advantage in looking younger, either as an age concealer (because it hides wrinkles) or as a visual signifier.	Some types of eyewear can make you look older.

CONTACT LENSES

Contact lenses are available for almost all powers of nearsightedness correction and for many in farsightedness. There are also contact lenses that can correct mild astigmatism. Also, old-age vision can be corrected by contact lenses. They work more or less in the same way as eyeglass lenses in a frame. The contact lenses have two powers in one lens, one to correct distance vision, if that's needed, and the other to correct near vision.

Having less correction in one of the contact lenses than is actually needed is called Monovision and this often means that you can avoid using reading glasses.

LASER SURGERY

Surgery has become a popular way of correcting eyesight. Surgery is fairly safe today, but as with all surgical procedures, there is always a risk. Therefore, carefully consider your options before deciding, and always consult an experienced ophthalmologist to do the procedure. There are several techniques available today. Avoid techniques that are still considered experimental (which some operations for farsightedness are).

GLASSES

Eyeglasses consist of a frame and two lenses. If you want to use glasses, you should be aware of the signals that frames and lenses give away.

Lenses

When choosing lenses, you have two options: plastic lenses or real-glass lenses. Plastic lenses weigh less than glass, are splinterless, and are less prone to dewing. They scratch easier, though some new plastic lenses that are hardened are less prone to scratches. Plastic lenses are thicker at higher powers, whereas regular glass is generally thinner than plastic at higher powers.

People who are nearsighted will typically also end up needing reading glasses. They will then need two different pairs of glasses—one pair for distance and one pair for reading. Or they can get one pair of glasses with lenses that correct for both near vision and presbyopia. There are two options for a combined lens: bifocals and multipower. You should always go for multipower. In bifocals, there is a rectangular area in the lenses that is used for reading. In bifocals, the reading area is very visible and reveals to others that the wearer needs reading glasses. In multipower lenses, the reading area is invisible. These lenses look just like regular glasses and will not reveal that the wearer needs reading glasses.

If you are nearsighted, thick lenses will make your eyes look smaller. If you are farsighted, thick lenses will make your eyes and everything under the lenses look bigger. This will include wrinkles.

Always make sure that you get anti-reflective coating on the lenses. This will ensure that both you and the frame look good.

Frames

The perception of glasses used to be that they made people look wiser—and also older. This is not the case anymore. Eyewear design has changed dramatically in recent years, and today eyewear has become an important accessory that can be used in different positive ways if you want to look younger. In fact, eyewear can be used to make anybody look younger, whether they need corrective lenses or not.

The right eyewear has several advantages. It can disguise wrinkles and send very youthful signals. The wrong kind of eyewear will do the exact opposite on both counts.

The most important thing is to avoid reading-glass-style eyewear, so-called half-frame eyewear. This kind of eyewear will reveal to all that here is a person who actually needs reading glasses because of aging. If you only need reading glasses, get a normal full frame with the power that you need for reading. You then use full-frame eyewear as reading glasses—they will just not look like reading glasses. Some people like half-frames because they do not have to take off the glasses when using their distance vision. With full-frames, you have to take the glasses off your nose when you're not reading. But this is the best solution with respect to camouflaging old-age vision.

EYEWEAR THAT HIDES WRINKLES

A pair of glasses can hide wrinkles around the eyes, and in some cases the eyewear can also take away attention from other parts of the face. In order to do so, you have to pay attention to the following parts of the frame:

- ❖ Size of frame
- ❖ Thickness of frame
- ❖ Placing and height of stems

Both too small and too large a frame will expose wrinkles around the eyes. Frames that are too large will also expose pouchy eyes. The thinness and thickness of the frame should be taken into consideration. Too thin a frame will not hide wrinkles.

The front of the frame is often what we pay most attention to when we choose eyewear. But the stems can also be effective in hiding wrinkles around the eyes, especially "crow's feet." Too thin a stem or a stem placed at the top of the front of the frame will not hide wrinkles. A stem that has some height will hide wrinkles.

The illustrations show variations as drawings, not real frames, on frame and stem height and placement. They show some principles but do not represent eyewear trends. However, it is important to be aware that eyewear not only can be used to conceal wrinkles, but also can be used as a visual signifier to signal youthfulness.

Too large a frame (left) and correct-sized frame to hide wrinkles

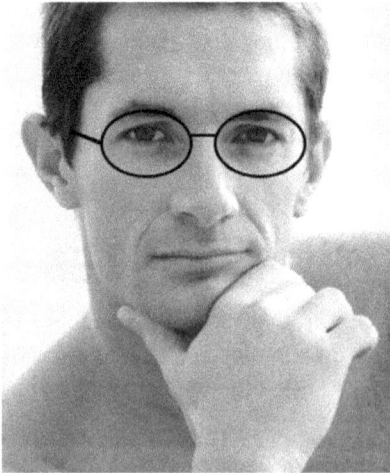

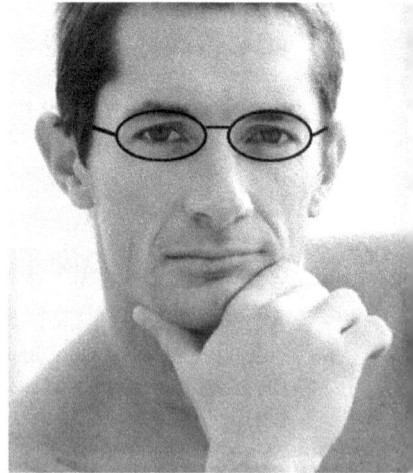

Too thin a frame (left) and a good frame
thickness to hide wrinkles

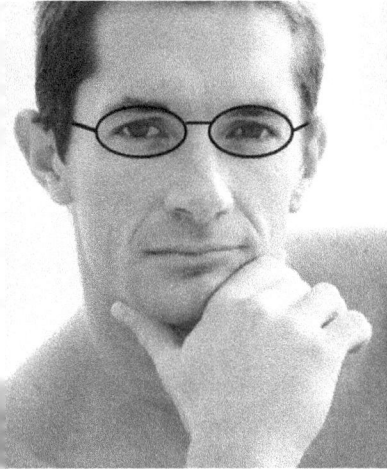

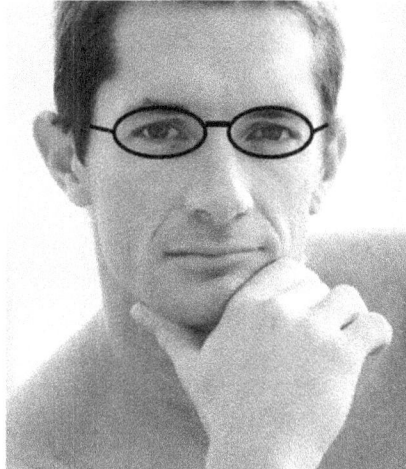

Stems that are too thin (left) and stems that are
correctly proportioned and placed to hide wrinkles

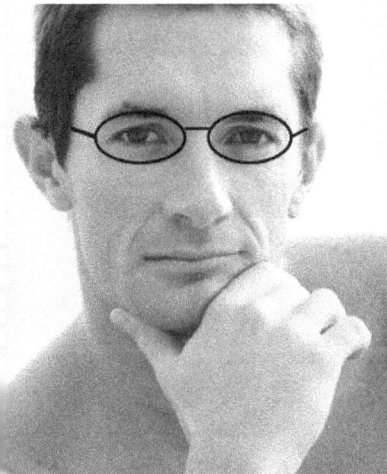

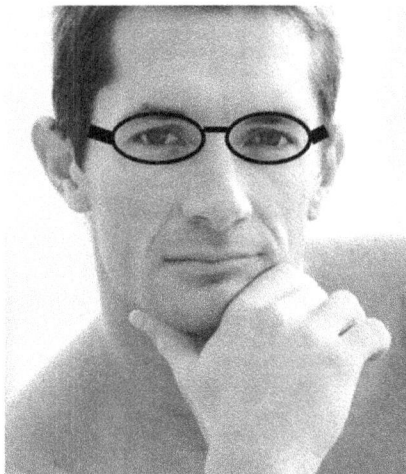

Age-Concealing Eyewear Selector Guide

Wrinkle Type	Eyewear Frame	Eyewear Color
Worry wrinkle	High nose bridge	Good match with eye color
Drooping eyebrow	Dominant upper frame	Same or similar color as eyebrows
Drooping eyelid	Small frame pointing up	Highlight eye color
Bags under the eyes	Small dominant frame	Highlight eye color
Dark circles under the eyes	Small dominant frame	Dark color

You can use eyewear whether you need prescription glasses or not. If you do not need prescription glasses, you can just have regular "window glass" as lenses.

Eyewear as Visual Signifier

Eyewear has become fashionable, and there are many trendy frames available in opticians' stores. If used properly, eyewear can be a very strong visual signifier. Eyewear is very visible—it is on the face—and if it is the right trendy eyewear, it will help communicate your desired visual age.

If you want a pair of glasses that can help you look younger, you can read men's fashion magazines. Many fashion magazines also keep you updated on eyewear trends.

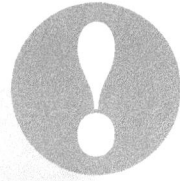

On your way to looking younger

❖ Consider carefully your options in contact lenses and/or eyewear if you need vision correction.

❖ Pay attention to eyewear that can make you look younger.

❖ Choose lenses with invisible power lines if you are both nearsighted and need reading glasses.

Youthful Hair for All

CHAPTER FOCUS
❖ Hair loss
❖ Hair color
❖ Hair styles

Many men are sensitive about how much hair they have—or don't have—on the top of their head. Some men start losing their hair and get a receding hairline when they are still in their twenties or thirties. No matter when it happens, balding is a typical male phenomenon that can cause men to look older. In most cases, there are options available that can both make a balding man feel good about himself and make him look the same age—or younger—as the guy who has all his hair. A bald head no longer signals a certain age because so many young men shave their head.

Without a doubt, hair is an important part of our appearance. Men who are not otherwise vain can act very vain when it comes to their hair. In some ways, it is even expected for men to be vain about their hair.

Hair holds many signals with respect to signaling our self-perceived age. But what we do with our hair has limitations compared to, say, clothing and accessories. The reason is the obvious one—that we do not ourselves control how much hair we have on our head as we grow older. This may limit the haircuts that we can choose. Even when we have all our hair, we can experience limitations because our hair type is not right for a certain haircut (it could be too thin, too curly, etc.). But the one major issue for many men is hair loss.

HAIR LOSS

Baldness is a biological process that happens to many men. Up to eighty percent of all men end up being affected by some sort of baldness. The cause for baldness is not fully understood. One theory is that baldness is caused by male hormones, and actually having the "right" levels of hormones for your age can accelerate hair loss (although this is probably not a comfort for the hormone-balanced men who would rather have all their hair).

Baldness is, in many cases, a sign of aging. Most men who are bald are in their fifties or older. But men in their twenties or thirties may start going bald, part of a biological process that has been "programmed" to happen because of the genetics inherited from previous generations.

Interestingly, our view of male baldness has changed a lot in the past couple of decades. There are many reasons for this:

❖ Short hair is the most popular hairstyle for men and has been so for quite some time.
❖ Very short hair is considered very masculine today—and to some people very short hair is very sexy.
❖ You didn't see balding men in movies for a long time in the twentieth century. Male movie stars always had all their hair. Some exceptions had a moderate receding A-shaped hairline. Now male movie stars can be balding in many different ways and still be thought of as attractive.

How other people react to bald or balding men depends upon how a man approaches his own baldness. One way it can be approached that will not make people think of baldness as an age-revealer is by shaving all the hair off.

Baldness comes in many different forms and shapes. Some types of baldness can be treated. But before a possible treatment can be found, you have to identify the type of balding that you are dealing with. Look in the Balding Patterns Overview chart to familiarize yourself with the kind of balding pattern that best describes your own balding pattern.

Balding Patterns Overview

Pattern	Characteristic
Thin-haired A-shape	Receding temples combined with thinning hair on top of head.
A-shaped receding hairline	Receding temples that do not affect hair on top of head but can be combined with a bald spot on top of head.
Thin-haired U-shape	Thinning hair on top of head but not at sides and on back of head.
U-shaped receding hairline	Hair receding from forehead and on top of head
Thin-haired bald spot	Hair on top of head is thinning
Bald spot	Spot on top of head without hair
Overall baldness	Either completely bald or with only a wreath of hair at back and at sides

When you have identified your balding pattern, go to the Hair Solutions Guide for Balding Men to get an overview of the possible solutions to your type of baldness.

Hair Solutions Guide for Balding Men

Options Balding pattern	Hair cut	Will medica-tion work for this type of baldness?	Surgery	Other options
Thin-haired receding A-shape*	Crew-cut	Yes	Micro grafts	Semi-crew-cut
A-shaped receding hairline, moderate*	Crew-cut	Maybe	Bald skin reduction	Longer hair swept back
A-shaped receding hairline, extensive*	Crew-cut	Not likely	Bald skin reduction	Complete shave
Thin-haired U-shape**	Complete shave	Yes	Micro grafts	Hairpiece
U-shaped receding hairline**	Complete shave	No	Micro grafts	Hairpiece
Bald upper forehead	Complete shave	No	Not recommended	Hairpiece
Thin-haired spot on top of head	Crew-cut	Yes	Yes	Weave
Bald spot	Crew-cut	No	Not recom-mended	Weave
Overall baldness	N/A	No	No	Wig

* There is hair on top of the head
** There is no hair on top of the head

Anti-hair Loss Medication

Throughout the years, all kinds of "wonder drugs" to give men their hair back have been marketed. No such drugs really exist, but today there are two medical treatment options available to treat hair loss. First came Minoxidil which, in some men, may cause increased growth. When the medication is discontinued, the hair loss returns to a normal rate within thirty to sixty days. Today, Minoxidil is sold under different brand names as a topical solution that is sprayed on the balding area. Minoxidil is not as effective when there is a large area of hair loss. In addition, its effectiveness has largely been demonstrated in men who have experienced hair loss for less than five years. Minoxidil is indicated for hair loss on top of the head only.

Now there is also another medication, Finasteride. This is a pill taken on a daily basis. Finasteride works on the top of the head. Studies have shown that two out of three men with mild to moderate hair loss who took Finasteride regrew some hair. Like Minoxidil, Finasteride is only effective while it is taken. The hair gained or maintained is lost within six to twelve months of stopping the medication.

Hair Surgery

Cosmetic plastic surgery may be an option for some balding men but should only be considered when the hair loss has been permanent for some time, at least five years. If you start surgery in an on-going process of hair loss, you have no guarantee what the result will be. There is a big risk that you will begin surgery thinking you know what the result will be—and instead you can end up having to fix what the surgery did in order not to look like someone who has had unsuccessful surgery. There is no official statistic of the number of men who are unhappy with the results of cosmetic hair surgery, but it is probably just as big as the number who are happy. Therefore, surgery takes a lot of consideration. You can get an overview of what types of baldness for which surgery is an option in the Surgical Procedures Selection Guide. You can get an impression of some of the pros and cons in the Surgical Procedures Options for Male Baldness Overview.

Surgical Procedures Selection Guide

Balding Pattern	Surgical Option
Thin-haired A-shape	Bald skin reduction
A-shaped receding hairline	Bald skin reduction
Thin-haired U-shape	Micro grafting
U-shaped receding hairline	Surgery not recommended
Thin-haired bald spot	Bald skin reduction or micro grafting
Bald spot	Bald skin reduction
Overall baldness	Surgery not recommended

Surgical Procedures Options for Male Baldness Overview

Treatment	Pros	Cons
Bald skin reduction (surgical removal of skin that does not grow hair any longer)	An option for men who are very unhappy with A-shaped receding hairline	If hair loss continues, there is a big risk for bald spots Thinner hair where hair is stretched Almost always leaves scarring General risks of infection
Micro grafting (surgical redistribution of single or two to four hair shafts; normally from back of head to top of head)	An option for men who are very unhappy with A-shaped or U-shaped receding hairlines	If hair loss continues, there is a big risk for very thin hair Leaves scarring on back of head Thinner hair on back of head General risks of infection
Hair transplant (surgical redistribution of large patches of hair follicles)	An option if other options are not possible	Leaves scarring on back of head Thinner hair on back of head General risks of infection

Anti-baldness Haircut Frequency Guidelines

With balding hair, it is very important to have frequent haircuts if you want to look less bald. Check the Anti-baldness Haircut Frequency Guidelines to find out how often different kinds of hairstyles need to be cut.

Hair style	Frequency
Shaved	Every second day
Crew-cut	Once a week
Semi-crew-cut	Every two weeks
Styled hair	Once a month
Longer-hair hair style	Once a month

NON-PERMANENT HAIR OPTIONS

More women than men use wigs and other kinds of hairpieces. On average, women have longer hair than men, and this makes it easier for women to hide the fact that they use a wig or hairpiece. And hiding is the whole point of wearing a wig or hairpiece. Men have three options: toupee, weave, and wig.

Toupee

A toupee is a hairpiece of natural or synthetic hair worn to cover partial baldness. Toupees are often custom made to the needs of the wearer, and can be manufactured using either synthetic or human hair. Toupées are usually held to one's head using an adhesive, which also means that they work best on a completely bald area.

Hair Weave

Hair weaves are a technique in which the toupee's base is woven into whatever natural hair the wearer retains. The toupee is attached to existing hair, often fairly tightly. Tightening of the weave should take place every four to five weeks to look natural. While hair weaves in principle may result in a less-detectable toupee, the wearer can experience discomfort and sometimes hair loss from frequently retightening the weave as one's own hair grows. After about six months, a person can begin to lose hair permanently along the weave area, resulting in so-called traction alopecia.

The jury is still out on hair weaving. Some men are happy with the result, though more are disappointed. There is a real risk of permanent hair damage, and hair loss must also be considered.

Pop singer Elton John has a hair weave, as do many other celebrities.

Wig

Whether you wear a toupee, weave, or wig is not what determines your age. It's the hairstyle or the style of the wig. The same style that signifies a certain age for real hair also applies to hairpieces and wigs.

Age-Specific Hairstyles

What visual age do you want to convey with your hairstyle? You may want to convey the same age as in clothing and accessories—or a slightly different age. Some men will want their hair to convey an age that is older than their visual age for clothing—and for other men, it will be the opposite. Again, study men's fashion magazines to get updated on men's hairstyles.

HAIR COLOR

Some people may have preferences for blonde, or brown, red, or black hair, but when it comes to hair color, specific hair colors do not convey certain ages. All hair colors can look equally young—except for gray or grayish hair. If you do not have gray or grayish hair, there is no age-related reason to dye your hair.

Gray or grayish hair is one of the biggest age revealers that we know. And getting graying hair happens to most people when they are old enough. But people can get gray hair at any age after thirty.

How early we start getting gray hair is determined by our genes. This means that most people will start getting gray hairs around the same age that their parents and grandparents first got their gray hair. From the time a person notices a few gray hairs, it may take more than ten years for all of that person's hair to turn gray. Gray hair is more noticeable in people with dark hair because it stands out, but people with light hair are just as likely to get gray hair.

The cause of gray hair is well known. The root of every strand of hair is fastened in a hair follicle. Each hair follicle contains a certain number of pigment cells (as does the skin). The pigment cells continuously produce a chemical called melanin (as does the skin) that gives growing hair its color of blonde, red, brown, black, etc. The dark or light color of someone's hair depends on how much melanin each hair contains.

As we get older, the pigment cells in the hair follicles gradually die. When there are fewer pigment cells in a hair follicle, the hair will no longer contain as much melanin and will become a more transparent color—like gray, silver, or white —as it grows. As we get older, there are fewer pigment cells to produce melanin. Eventually, the hair will be completely gray.

Luckily, gray hair is also one of the easiest hair issues to do something about—with hair dye. Use the Age-Concealing Hair-Dyeing Guidelines for the best results. If you have gray or grayish dyed hair, you should consider dyeing your hair into your own original hair color or get a salt-and-pepper color.

Age-Concealing Hair-Dyeing Guidelines

1. It is important that dyed hair does not *look* like dyed hair. What's the point in dyeing your hair to conceal your age if the dyeing shows the world that you dye your hair and reveals that maybe you need to dye your hair to conceal your age?

2. If hair and skin tone match the dyed hair, you will look the most natural. If you stick to your original hair color, you can be sure that hair and skin color match.

3. If you are in doubt about the natural color of your hair, use the online Skin Tone and Hair Color Matching Guide online.

4. If all hair is dyed the same color, the hair can look dyed. Make sure that there is natural tone to your dyed hair. This can be done by using a multi-color kit. This will contain a brush like a mascara brush that can be used to create different nuances in the hair.

5. Touch-up the dye when new gray hair appears from the roots.

Skin Tone and Hair Color Matching Guide

Generally, the hair color should only be one to three shades different from the skin tone. If in doubt about the natural color of your hair, you can use the Skin Tone and Hair Color Matching Guide, which (in grey tones) tell you that the darker the skin tone, the darker hair color will look natural.

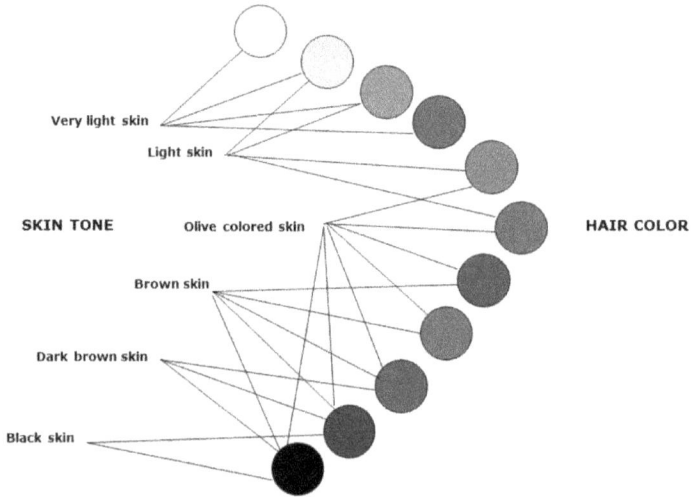

Very light skin
Light skin

SKIN TONE Olive colored skin **HAIR COLOR**

Brown skin

Dark brown skin

Black skin

Hearing Aids

For some people, a loss of hearing is part of growing old. About fifteen percent of people between the biological ages of sixty and eighty will have some kind of hearing loss. For some, the reduction of hearing will warrant a hearing aid early in life, but for most people a hearing aid is only needed late in life. If a hearing aid is warranted, you will want to conceal it, of course. Technology has changed the shape and the design of hearing aids dramatically since the beginning of the twenty-first century. Today, there are many options, and the right hearing aids for people who want to look younger are miniscule and hidden inside the ear. Otherwise, hairstyle plays an important role in hiding a hearing aid.

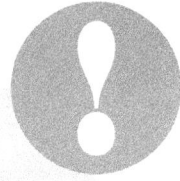

On your way to looking younger

❖ When partially bald or balding, shave off the remaining hair

❖ For some men, medical treatment options will stop hair loss or regrow hair

❖ Trim or cut short hair frequently

Facial Hair or Not?

CHAPTER FOCUS

❖ Facial hair overview
❖ Beards
❖ Face piercings

As we age, changes happen to our face. First, we see changes in the skin. Later, we may experience changes in our eyebrows and other facial hair. The eyebrow hairs may grow longer, and like the hair on the top of the head, the color of facial hair may also turn grey. All this means that we have to be aware that facial hair sends signals about our age. So when a man wants to look younger, this is one of the areas where a lot can be gained, often with very little effort.

When we look for signs of aging, we tend to look at the face, and with good reason. The face is the part of our body that we ourselves look at the most. We look at our hair (it may be thinning or turning grey) and we look at the skin (eventually we see wrinkles). When young, we do not tend to pay a lot of attention to our facial hair unless we have a beard and/or sideburns.

When we have a beard or sideburns, it can be a matter of personal style or fashion. The latter is often the case for men. As with so many other things that have an element of fashion at different times in history, beards and moustaches have fallen in and out of fashion. Whenever beards are popular with young men, it certainly makes sense to imitate them and have the same style of beard they have—unless the beard will be grey. Of course, a man can have a grey beard, and he should if that is what he wants. But a grey beard is a big age-revealer, so if the point is to look younger, you should drop the beard. A clean-shaven face is preferred.

Even if your beard is not grey, you should be aware that beards almost always make you look older. Up to a certain age, say forty, you should not worry about a beard making you look older. But beards on men past forty can sometimes make the man look ten or more years older just by having the beard.

What goes for beards also goes for sideburns. Your sideburns may turn grey before the hair on the top of your head. If that is the case, you should drop the sideburns or dye them to match.

All facial hair can turn grey. This also includes the eyebrows. We can decide not to have a beard and sideburns, but we cannot decide not to have eyebrows. So our eyebrows should get some extra attention when we begin to see changes in them. One of the first changes we see in eyebrows is typically extra hair growth. Later, there may be a change in color, often to grey or white. At first a few hairs will change color and then more than a few.

One interesting thing is that a man is very rarely considered vain when he takes care of his facial hair. That is, of course, the way it should be. This means that there is carte blanche to do what it takes to look younger with respect to grooming your facial hair.

The Facial Hair Overview is a list of all types of facial hair. In this list, you can see if the hair type has influence on our age-related appearance.

Facial Hair Overview

Facial hair type	Influence on age-related appearance?
Sideburns	Yes
Beards	Yes
Eyebrows	Yes
Eyelashes	No
Ear hair	Yes
Nose hair	Yes

In the Look Younger Facial Hair Adjustment Guidelines, there are suggestions on what to do in order to change the age-revealing signals that facial hair has.

Look Younger Facial Hair Adjustment Guidelines

Facial hair type	Suggested adjustment(s)
Sideburns	If grey ❖ Shave them off ❖ Trim them ❖ Color them if you color your hair
Beard	If grey, do not grow a beard
Eyebrows	Remove long hairs; reduce if bushy (learn more later in this chapter)
Eyelashes	Leave them as they are
Ear hair	Remove all hair in ears regularly
Nose hair	Remove all hair in nose regularly

Use the Hair Removing Techniques and Tools Guide to find out about the techniques and tools you have at your disposal if you want to reduce facial hair.

Hair Removing Techniques and Tools Guide

Hair removal technique/tool	Where generally used by men
Shaving with electric razor	Beard, sideburns
Shaving with razor	Beard, sideburns
Trimming with hair trimmer	Beard, sideburns
Nose hair trimmer	Use to remove hair from nose and in ears
Scissors	Can be used to cut eyebrow hair if eyebrow is very bushy. See section on eyebrows.
Pincers	Use to remove long hairs from eyebrows. See section on eyebrows. Use to remove stray hairs all over the face.

Avoid the Uneven Shave

With age, most people need reading glasses. But some people also need them for other daily activities. Among them is shaving. You actually may need glasses for shaving before you need them for reading. When we read, we can extend our arms further and further away from our eyes. But when shaving while standing in front of the mirror, we don't really have the same option. Good light and a proper shaving mirror can help us see if there are any hairs left on the face and neck. But at some point that will not be enough.

With perfect eyesight, we can easily see when we are done shaving all beard hairs off and are truly clean-shaven. But with the changes in eyesight, it becomes difficult to really see if there are small hairs left on the face. Some beard hairs we may be able to feel by touching, but that is not possible with very short hairs. Sometimes it is the long, single stray hairs that can be difficult to see with reduced eyesight.

An uneven shave is a big age-revealer because we typically see an uneven shave on the faces of men who are older—and only on men who need glasses and do not use them. So glasses are an important tool with respect to shaving. You can read more about glasses in Chapter 8.

EYEBROW SPECIAL

Eyebrows can have different shapes. They can be thin, thick, nicely shaped, or some sort of unibrow (when the two eyebrows grow together). How the eyebrow looks from nature has no influence on how old you look. It is only when you see changes in your eyebrow that you should start paying attention to them. The changes typically start when a man is in his late forties.

The change can be about the number of hairs, their length, and/or their color. Often a change starts with the appearance of some stray hairs (that are easy to get rid of). In the Eyebrow Changes Overview, you can see a list of some typical changes that can happen to men's eyebrows.

Eyebrow Changes Overview

Look of eyebrow	What to do
Some stray hairs (long, thick, or white) once in a while	Use a pair of pincers to remove the individual hairs. See more in the DIY section below.
Stray hairs on a regular basis	Use a pair of pincers to remove the individual hairs. See more in the DIY section below.
Many thick and stiff hairs	Use a pair of pincers to remove the individual hairs or get help from a salon specialist.
Many long hairs	Use a small pair of scissors to cut long hairs. Avoid cutting other hairs.
Bushy hairs	Use a small pair of scissors to cut bushy hair. Try to cut small sections of the eyebrow at a time so that all hairs are not cut evenly. Consider getting help from a salon specialist.
Many white or grey hairs	See section on coloring.
Combinations of the above	Use a combination of methods or go to a salon specialist.

DIY or Salon?

If you don't mind standing in front of the mirror using a pair of pincers on your eyebrows, you can remove stray hairs yourself. You may even be able to handle a pair of scissors yourself if you need to cut long hairs or very bushy eyebrows. If it does not work for you on your own, get someone you know to do it for you or get a professional specialist at a hair salon or a cosmetologist, maybe at a day spa.

You may feel hesitant about going to a professional specialist; maybe you feel a little embarrassed that you need help or you are worried you will be considered vain. First of all, people who work as hair dressers or cosmetologists will never find it embarrassing that you need their professional help. And vanity is their business. They are likely to think that vanity is a very good thing.

How do you find the right professional? Ask your hairdresser if he or she does eyebrows or knows someone who does. Otherwise, you can check the yellow pages, newspaper advertisements, or online.

When you choose a specialist, it is important that you choose one who does men's eyebrows on a regular basis because men's eyebrows should be treated in a different way from women's eyebrows. A woman's eyebrow can be styled or shaped in a different way than what is natural. A man's eyebrow should never look styled or plucked. It should look completely natural, as if it has not been touched by a human hand, so to speak. If you get help from a specialist, stress again and again that you want the result to look completely natural. You want to keep the shape and look of your eyebrow the way it was when you were in your thirties.

Your idea of what is natural and what a professional thinks is natural can be two completely different things. Therefore, follow these guidelines:

❖ Ask that hair be removed with the threading technique or with a pair of pincers. (The threading technique is described below.) This allows for individual unwanted hairs to be removed without removing hair that you want to keep.
❖ Ask that all the fine, almost invisible hair around the actual eyebrow is NOT removed. If these hairs are removed, your eyebrow will look styled.
❖ Say no to having your eyebrow waxed. It will remove all the fine, almost invisible hair. (You can read about waxing in the next chapter.)

❖ Ask that only stray hairs, extra-long hairs, thick hairs, bushy hairs, and white or grey hairs be removed, preferably one by one, so that only the unwanted hairs are removed. If your eyebrow only consists of white or grey hairs, have only stray hairs removed. If your *hair* is not white or grey, you may consider having your eyebrows colored. (See more on this at the end of this chapter.)

❖ Hesitate to have scissors used. If scissors are used, all hairs will be cut evenly, which shows that something has been done to your eyebrows. Only if you have very bushy eyebrows or you have many long hairs should scissors be used.

❖ You may be told that it will be faster and cheaper to use wax or scissors. Do not budge. This is an area where you should not save money.

❖ Stress again and again that you want a completely natural-looking result, that is, your eyebrows should look the way they have always looked.

Threading

Threading is a hair removal technique where a thin cotton thread is used as a sort of mini lasso around an unwanted hair (or sometimes more hairs). When the hair is trapped, it is pulled out of the hair follicle. An experienced cosmetologist can thread hairs very precisely. It is not something that you can do yourself.

DIY Step-by-Step

Use this step-by-step guide if you are just beginning to see changes in your eyebrows.

1. Get in front of a mirror with lots of light. It is a good idea to use a shaving mirror.
2. Use a pair of pincers (not too pointed and not too wide).
3. Remove any obvious stray hairs from the eyebrow.
4. Remove any obvious white or grey hairs.
5. With your finger, press all eyebrow hairs against their natural growth direction. Any very long hairs will be easily identifiable.
6. Remove any extra-long hairs.
7. Smooth hair back to natural position.
8. How does it look? Double check that you have removed all unwanted hair.

COLORING

In principle, it is possible to color facial hair. But there are some buts with respect to coloring facial hair. First of all, it must look natural. Facial hair can easily look colored, which will reveal that you color your facial hair. This is age-revealing. Just as with hair coloring on the head, coloring of facial hair should look as natural as possible. However, if you are dark haired or color your hair dark, it will make sense to have sideburns, eyelashes, and eyebrows match the color of your hair.

It is very, very rare for a man to color his beard, and it is not recommended. Drop the beard instead. If you color your hair, then sideburns can also be colored in the same color, but it does not always give the natural look that is desired. It is better to simply not have sideburns.

Unless your hair is completely black, never have eyelashes or eyebrows colored black. It will look artificial. Eyelashes should be dark brown (or lighter depending on hair color). Eyebrows should match the color of sideburns.

Facial hair will grow back to its natural color. This takes as long a time as it takes for the hair to grow. On eyebrows and eyelashes, colored hair will fall off and be replaced with new, non-colored hair. This normally takes one to two months to happen.

There are Do-It-Yourself toolkits to color eyebrows and eyelashes. But it is not recommended that you do it yourself. This is one situation where you should go to a salon and get a professional to do the coloring. Underline again and again that you want a natural look.

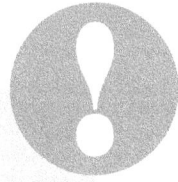

On your way to looking younger

❖ Drop your beard and sideburns if you have grey hair

❖ Be extra meticulous with your eyebrows

❖ Drop face piercings

CHAPTER 11

The Matter of Body Hair

- ❖ Body hair overview
- ❖ Hair removal
- ❖ Tattoos

To many people—both men and women—body hair on a man is the essence of masculinity. But young men, in particular, have begun removing hair from their upper body, and this affects other men. Now hair on the body has simply lost some of its masculine significance, and all men can signal youthfulness by not having (a lot of) hair on their upper body. Shaving off hair does not equal shaving off masculinity. Now we know that you can be just as masculine as the next man when you shave some or all hair off the upper body.

TO BE OR NOT TO BE—HAIRY

Once upon a time (in the 1900s), hair on the chest was considered very manly. No man would think of shaving off his chest hair. But sometime around the beginning of the new century, the thinking on body hair changed dramatically. More and more men started to shave their chests (and other parts of their body). In the course of a decade, we got a new male beauty ideal. What happened?

Many men have become more physically active in their spare time. In recent decades, the number of men who go to the gym or do other kinds of sports has exploded. Gyms were originally the favoured domain of bodybuilders, and among bodybuilders it has always been popular to shave all hair off the body in order to clearly see the muscle definition on the chest and stomach. Now that gyms are for everybody, this behaviour has become mainstream. Even if you work out in a gym and do not necessarily have a lot of muscles, you can, like more and more men, especially young men, shave off your body hair.

Actually, men shaving off their body hair does not just happen in the gym. Many athletes, in particular swimmers, have been shaving off their body hair for decades. Tour de France cyclists are known for shaving their arms and legs. Soccer players also shave their legs because they are prone to skin injuries, and wounds are quicker to treat if there is no hair, and there is less risk of infection. Triathlon is a popular extreme sport consisting of swimming, biking, and running, and triathletes shave off all or some of their body hair. So a growing group of men realize that when top athletes can shave off their body hair, so can they.

We can call it a new male beauty ideal or whatever we feel like, but basically this is what this book is about, looking younger. Both men and women see that *young* men do not have chest hair (or not a lot of it), and men of any age who want to look younger simply have to follow suit. Now the thinking is that a lot of hair on the body makes a man look older, and, of course, as he gets older this hair will be grey. And grey hair—whether on the top of the head or on the body— holds the same signals about age (that you are past a certain age).

But why think about hair on the body (grey or any color) if you stay fully clothed most of the year? Well, shaving off your chest hair can have symbolic meaning. When shaving off your chest hair, you are symbolically removing age from your body. Sometimes we underestimate the influence our thoughts have on how we feel with respect to age. And though most of us are fully clothed most of the day, we do take showers, undress to go to bed, have sex, go to the gym, or do other types of physical exercise, and we are then confronted with our naked body. We want to see a young-looking body when we purposely or by chance look in the mirror because this affects how we think of ourselves. How we think of ourselves is directly linked to what we see in the mirror. When we look in the (full body) mirror and see a man that looks younger than his biological age, we are pleased.

So a shaved chest is not just about an aesthetic ideal, it is about wellbeing on several levels.

More and more men also remove hair in the pubic area. Typically, all the hair on the testicles and maybe some of the hair around the penis is removed. As with all hair removal, it is something that can be observed when we go to the gym. From there, it is talked about among both men and women (men tell their wives or girlfriends who tell their female friends about it). It may be done for aesthetic, hygienic, or sexual reasons, and it may be done for oneself or for one's partner's sake. So while this can hardly be said to have much to do with looking younger, it is behaviour mostly observed among young men, and thus has symbolic value, if only to oneself and one's partner.

Body hair is not just about chest hair and pubic hair. The Body Hair Overview is a list of all types of body hair. In this list, you can see if the hair type has influence on our age-related appearance.

Body Hair Overview

Hair type	Influence on age-related appearance?
Chest hair	Yes
Hair on stomach	Yes
Hair in armpits	No
Hair on back and shoulders	Yes
Pubic hair	Some
Hair on arms	No
Hair on hands/fingers	No
Hair on legs	No
Hair on feet and toes	No

In the Look Younger Body Hair Adjustment Guidelines, there are suggestions on what to do to change the age-revealing signals that hair has.

Look Younger Body Hair Adjustment Guidelines

Hair type	Suggested adjustment(s)
Chest hair	Trim hair or remove hair. Trimmed hair should be about a quarter of an inch.
Hair on stomach	Remove hair from stomach area.
Hair in armpits	Should only be reduced if you are bothered by amount of hair or for hygienic reasons.
Hair on back and shoulders	Remove hair. You can get razors that are extra long so that they can reach onto your back. Many men go to a salon to have hair on the back removed.
Hair on arms	Should only be removed/reduced if you are bothered by amount of hair or color of hair.
Hair on hands/fingers	Should only be removed/reduced if you are bothered by amount of hair or color of hair.
Hair on legs	Should only be removed/reduced if you are bothered by amount of hair or color of hair.
Hair on feet and toes	Should only be removed/reduced if you are bothered by amount of hair or color of hair.
Pubic hair	Some men remove hair on testicles and around the penis for hygienic or other reasons.

Use the Hair Removing Techniques and Tools Guide to find out the techniques and tools you have at your disposal if you want to reduce body hair.

Hair Removing Techniques and Tools Guide

Hair removal technique/tool	Effect	Where generally used by men
Shaving with electric razor	Up to 2 weeks	All over body (except intimate areas)
Shaving with razor	Up to 2 weeks	All over body
Trimming with hair trimmer	1 to 2 weeks	Chest hair and hair on stomach
Cream/gel	Up to 1 month	All over body
Waxing	Up to 2 months	Mostly used on back and shoulders (should be done by a professional in a salon)
Electrolysis	Permanent	In principle, all over the body
Laser	Semi-permanent	In principle, all over the body

Hair Removal Creams and Gels

Hair removal creams and gels are available. They are easy to use, even in the shower. They offer a painless and quick (usually less than five minutes) solution. Hair removal creams and gels can be used all over the body, but be careful to follow instructions. Areas of use may vary from brand to brand. Some may not be suitable for areas with sensitive skin, for instance, the testicles.

Waxing

Waxing is a form of hair removal that removes the unwanted hair from the root. New hair will normally not grow back in the waxed area for one to two months. Almost any area of the body can be waxed, including legs, arms, back, abdomen, and feet. There are many types of waxing suitable for removing unwanted hair.

Strip waxing is the most popular form of waxing. It is accomplished by spreading a thin layer of wax over the skin. A cloth or paper strip is then pressed on the top and ripped off in the direction of hair growth. This removes the wax along with the hair.

Hot waxing is another common form of waxing. In this case, the wax is applied somewhat thickly and with no cloth or paper strips. The wax hardens when it cools, thus allowing the easy removal without the aid of cloths.

Waxing should be carried out by an experienced cosmetologist.

Electrolysis

Electrolysis is the process of removing hair permanently by sliding a solid hair-thin metal probe into each hair follicle. Proper insertion does not puncture the skin.

Electricity is delivered to the follicle through the probe, which causes localized damage to the area that generates hair, so that a new hair will not grow out again from that follicle. The power and duration of the electricity are started at the lowest setting, then gradually increased until the hair comes out as easily as possible.

Depending on how much hair a client wants removed, the process can take from weeks to years. Electrolysis should be carried out by a certified professional.

Laser

Laser hair removal is the process of removing unwanted hair by means of exposure to pulses of laser light that destroy the hair follicle.

Hair grows in several phases, and a laser can only affect the active growing hair follicles. Therefore, several sessions are needed to kill hair in all phases of growth. Normally a waiting period from three to eight weeks between sessions is recommended. The number of sessions depends on which area of the body is being treated, skin color, and coarseness of hair. Laser does not work well on light-colored hair, red hair, grey hair, white hair, as well as fine hair of any color. Coarse dark hair on light skin is easiest to treat.

Laser hair removal should be carried out by a certified professional.

Tattoos

For decades, tattoos were in the sole domain of men, in particular, sailors and bikers. In the 1990s, tattoos became more widespread among men, and also among women. In particular, many young women got a small tattoo. It might be on the back, on the shoulder, or at the ankle. Though tattoos have been popular with the young age groups, this does not mean that the rest of the world interprets tattoos as young or youthful, at least not when it comes to women. Tattoos are also trendy, and because style changes, it is often best to avoid something as permanent as a tattoo.

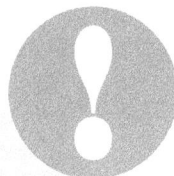

On your way to looking younger

❖ Remove or trim chest hair

❖ Remove stomach hair

❖ Don't get tattoos in order to look younger

12

Fragrances for Any Age

CHAPTER FOCUS
❖ Trendy fragrances
❖ Age-specific fragrances

Has fragrance anything to do with how young we look? No and yes. Fragrance has something to do with how youthful we *smell*. As there are also trends in fragrance, a fragrance can be used to highlight the signals we are sending with our clothes, accessories, hair, etc. Using the fragrance guide in this chapter, you have a chance to find a fragrance that will underline—and not undermine—your desired visual age.

Movies, magazines, and television cannot tell us how the young people we watch or read about smell. But as fragrance has become so common to use, there is no doubt that fragrance plays an important part in the signals we send. And as with other items that contain an element of style and taste, there are different choices, and some fragrances will be preferred by certain age groups. If we can identify the preferred fragrances for each age group, we have one more tool at our disposal when we want to radiate youthfulness.

Fragrance Basics

Fragrances are typically categorized into these six groups:

Citrus: Scents from citrus fruits, such as lime, lemon, tangerine, and mandarin. These are refreshing and light.

Green: Grassy scents with pine, juniper, and leaves. Have a sporty aroma.

Mossy: A combination of fresh herbs and mossy ferns. Have a strong and fresh aroma.

Woodsy: A notably woodsy-mossy mix with hints of bergamot, oak moss, and patchouli. Have a sweet and earthy aroma.

Floral: Scents from flowers, such as roses, orange blossoms, gardenias, jasmine, and carnations. The smell is like standing in a floral boutique.

Oriental: A mix of spices, amber, balsams, and resins. Has a heavy, musky scent.

Trends in fragrance change just as trends in fashion do. In the 1990s, citrus became very popular and was what young people preferred. Later heavy oriental aromas become popular. The heavy, oriental aromas are the opposite of the citrus scent, which meant that in the 1990s, this scent was not youthful at all.

The length of time the fragrance has been on the market often plays a part in how trendy it is. Some people fall in love with certain fragrances when they are first introduced and buy them again and again, even for decades if the particular fragrance is still available. Therefore, fragrances that have been on the market for years will often be preferred by older people, whereas new fragrances may be just getting their following among young people who may become fans for life, just as older people have become fans with the older fragrances.

The Fragrance Guide has suggestions for fragrances for five different age groups.

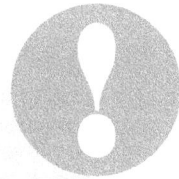

On your way to looking younger

❖ Fragrances can be used to send signals about age.

❖ Avoid fragrances that have been on the market for decades.

CHAPTER 13

Lifestyle Accessories

CHAPTER FOCUS

❖ Cell phones
❖ Cameras
❖ Music players
❖ Laptops
❖ Luggage

More and more objects are not only about functionality but also about style. When style becomes part of a product category, we start interpreting the design as we do with fashion—something that sends out different signals, including the age of the person using the products. This means that you have to pay attention to the style of the products that you use. Some products are perceived as more youthful than others are. Here is an overview of product categories where style plays a role.

Most people are not aware of it, but today we have more possibilities of signifying youthfulness than ever before because of the so-called lifestyle accessories. The term "accessory" is changing; rather, what are considered accessories is changing. There are the traditional accessories, such as sunglasses, bags, and shoes. Now there are also lifestyle accessories, for instance, cell phones, music players, and suitcases. These are designed products that can also be used to send youthful signals.

There are many different types of products to choose from in the lifestyle categories. Identifying the products that are appealing to young people is partly about identifying what is new and innovative, but it's not only that. There are many reasons for certain preferences in lifestyle products, and some have to do with how young people live their lives. But anybody who wants to underline their youthfulness can use lifestyle products, as long as they choose the right ones.

Though they are not as age-specific as other accessories, there certainly are some lifestyle accessories that work better than others. Here is an overview of five different lifestyle accessories categories that are heavily influenced by style:

Cell Phones
More and more people are using cell phones, and there are many to choose from. This means that it is important to choose a model that has a stylish and innovative look.

Tablet computers
If you use a computer, there are many to choose from, not least of which is the portable kind. Many people also use a tablet computer. They, too, can convey some powerful, youthful signals.

Luggage
Luggage with wheels is very practical and is why people of a certain age started using suitcases and carry-ons with wheels. Now, everybody is using luggage with wheels simply because it makes traveling so much easier. But it is important to choose, for instance, trolleys that do not make you appear any older than you are.

Fashion magazines will often also report on lifestyle accessories.

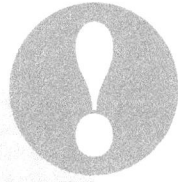

On your way to looking younger

❖ If you use lifestyle accessories, be aware that they also signal age.

❖ Choose lifestyle accessories that are fairly new to the market.

❖ If you want to use lifestyle accessories to help underline your desired visual age, you have to change them at certain intervals.

Cues for the Young Mind

CHAPTER FOCUS

❖ Personality
❖ Life phases
❖ Music
❖ Books
❖ Movies

With all the effort you put into looking younger than your biological age, why not also nourish a youthful mind? It is worth remembering that, to some people, it is the age of the mind that truly reveals a person's age. To take advantage of this, we have to be aware that our interests and conversations change as we grow older; make sure that you can share interests and conversation not only with people your own age but also with people whose biological age matches your self-perceived age.

Our body and face change as we age, but there is one thing that does not change—our personality. Psychological research has documented that the basic traits in our personality do not change a lot over time.

Our personality is, to a great extent, fully developed by our early twenties. If, at twenty, you are extroverted and speak rapidly, you are likely to be the same at seventy. And if you are modest and insecure when you are twenty, then it is not very likely that this will have changed when you are forty.

So, while our looks change as we age, we have a stable core inside—our personality—that is not likely to change dramatically once it is fully developed. This is the conclusion drawn from a number of studies in which scientists have observed the same group of people for several decades. In several of the studies, more than thirty years passed between the first and the last personality tests.

PERSONALITY AND AGE

One study was begun in the 1930s. Back then, a group of high school students was interviewed for a long-term study of personality traits. When they were twenty years old, they were interviewed a second time. The third interview took place when they were in their mid-thirties, and the final one when they were forty-five years old. During each interview, they were asked about their attitudes towards life, and, depending on the subject's age, parents, teachers, or spouses were also interviewed about the subject's personality at that particular time in his or her life.

Clinical psychologists made personality charts for each individual and continually analyzed the results. The scientists tested ninety different character traits for each subject, and in all cases there was a close personality resemblance between individual subjects in high school and the same person three decades later. Lively and optimistic teenagers had the same positive attitude in their forties. And individuals who had been very moody in high school were just as moody as adults.

In another study, psychologists from the National Institute of Aging in Baltimore, Maryland, studied several hundred men from the time they were about twenty-five years old until they retired. Based on the subjects' responses to a number of hypotheses and questions, they were placed in different categories: insecure, anxiety-prone, co-dependent, etc. This study confirmed the hypothesis that the personality an individual exhibits in his or her early twenties will not change for the rest of his or her life.

Another study of personalities focused on middle-aged and elderly people. Back in 1947, scientists at the University of Minnesota tested seventy-one men in their fifties. Thirty years later, the same group of men was tested again. The conclusion: their personality traits had not changed. There was, for instance, no change in the degree of extroversion and introversion during the thirty-year time period. The fifty-year-olds who had been sociable and self-assured had precisely the same traits when they were eighty.

OUR PERSONALITY DOES NOT CHANGE WITH AGE

In another study from the University of California at Berkeley, the researchers were interested in studying the development in women's personalities over time. A group of psychologists interviewed fifty-three women when they were thirty years old, and again when they were seventy years old. This study confirmed the other studies: there were no changes in, for instance, extroversion, irritability, or happiness. Women who were grumblers when they were thirty were grumblers throughout their adult life.

Few psychologists will conclude that no changes take place in personality over time for all people—it is just not the norm. Illness, such as depression, can have an enormous influence on one's personality, as can stressful situations, such as unemployment, divorce, or the death of a close family member. But there is a difference between short-lived changes in behavior and personality and fundamental and definitive changes in personality.

This is good news for all who are happy about their personality (or whose family and friends are happy with it). Some things do not change, and we do not have to worry about an "aging personality."

The studies do not claim that people do not change at all psychologically. It is only natural that our needs, interests, and attitudes change with age. That change often seems to go in a certain direction—we become more conservative. Not necessarily in the political sense of the word, but in the sense that we have "figured everything out" and maybe we are not as flexible in our needs, interests, and attitudes as we used to be.

Being conservative in the non-political sense of the word can be quite counterproductive to a youthful image. The young mind is—generally speaking—more open-minded, curious, and excited by new things (of all kinds). A person who is open-minded, curious, and excited by new things, therefore, will underline youthful signals.

The consequence is not a change in your personality (which is not really an option, anyway). But people will perceive you as being younger if you are able to relate to topics and issues that people younger than you relate to or are interested in. Then people who are younger than you will be interested in talking to you and hearing your opinion. Being associated with people who are younger than you—in one way or another—will also reflect on you and make you appear younger, too.

A young mind—no matter the biological age of the mind—is curious about many things. It is not about changing one's own preferences and dislikes but being aware that there are other tastes—and being open-minded to other people's tastes.

You can learn a little bit or have your memory refreshed by listening to music, reading books, and/or seeing movies that young people are interested in or that describe what it is like to be young.

AGE-SPECIFIC MUSIC GENRES

One thing that is a big age revealer is music. The older generation generally does not like the music that young people like. This has been the situation for decades and is not likely to change. But the generations' taste in music does change. Music changes all the time—a fact that can spark many discussions between the generations about musical taste.

There is no doubt that some people who listened to a certain kind of music when they were young will continue to like this music for many years. Others will move on to other kinds of music. This gives a very mixed picture of musical tastes. But there are some music genres different age groups listen to. You can get an overview of the most popular genres in the Age-specific Music Genre Guide.

Age-specific Music Genre Guide

Age group Music Genre	20s	30s	40s	50s	60s
New Age		X	X	X	
Electronica		X	X		
Dance music	X	X			
House	X	X			
Hip-hop & Rap	X	X			
R 'n' B	X	X			
Soul		X	X	X	X
Blues			X	X	X
Pop	X	X	X		
Evergreens				X	X
Easy Listening			X	X	X
Latin Music	X	X	X	X	X
Classic Rock			X	X	X
Modern Rock	X	X	X		
Hard Rock & Metal	X	X			
Folk		X	X	X	X
Country	X	X	X	X	X
Jazz				X	X
Classical			X	X	X
Opera			X	X	X
Musicals			X	X	X

You do not have to become a lover or an expert of any music that you do not like in order to convey a youthful mind. It seems that many people have great difficulty in acknowledging music that they don't like. But being aware and acknowledging that there are types of music that certain age groups like—and which are different from your own personal taste—is a big step in communicating across generations. You can use the Age-specific Music Genre Guide to establish which music genres you like and find out if there are some other genres that are close to your taste—but more youthful—that may be worth getting to know better.

LITERARY STIMULATION FOR YOUTHFUL MINDS

A youthful mind is curious and open-minded. You can test whether this is the case for your mind with five books about youth and about being young.

Jack Kerouac:
On the Road
Jack Kerouac's classic novel that defined a generation. On the Road is the quintessential American vision of freedom and hope, a book that changed American literature and changed anyone who has ever picked it up.

John Updike:
Run, Rabbit
Harry "Rabbit" Angstrom was a high school superstar only a handful of years ago. Now he is a young married father, trapped in the suburban sixties, unhappy with a cluttered house, a drunken wife, and a son who will never be the athlete he was. Will this former basketball star find a way to make his life better, or will he run like a rabbit? The title says it all.

J.D. Salinger:
Catcher in the Rye

The story of a couple of days in a sixteen-year-old boy's life just after he's been expelled from prep school; with his constant wry observations about what he encounters, from teachers to other phonies, the book captures the essence of the eternal teenage experience of alienation. One of the most important books to come out of the twentieth century.

Sue Townsend:
The Secret Diary of Adrian Mole, Aged 13 3/4

Teen angst has never been such serious business—or this much fun. In his secret diary, teen Adrian Mole excruciatingly details every morsel of his turbulent adolescence. Mixed in with daily reports about the zit sprouting on his chin are heartrending passages about his parents' chaotic marriage. Adrian sees all, and he has something to say about everything.

Mark Salzman:
The Laughing Sutra

This is what *Washington Post Book World* wrote about this book: "A rich blend of fantasy, philosophy, history and romance. Salzman is a master storyteller and the fortunate reader will find himself entranced, entertained, and very definitely enlightened."

ENTERTAINMENT FOR
YOUTHFUL MINDS

Ten memorable movies about *being* young—in case you need to refresh your memory.

The Graduate

Graduating from college, and then what? Recent college graduate Benjamin Braddock starts an affair with Mrs. Robinson, the wife of his father's neighbor and business partner, and then finds himself falling in love with her teenage daughter, Elaine.

American Graffiti

A couple of high school grads are scheduled to leave for college in the morning. Each has his own doubts about his future. They spend a final evening cruising the strip with their buddies and have every adventure possible before dawn when they will each have to decide what they will do.

Almost Famous

William Miller is a fifteen-year-old boy, hired by *Rolling Stone* magazine to tour with, and write about, an up-and-coming rock band. This authentic coming-of-age film follows William as he falls face first while confronting life, love, and lingo.

Grease

Good girl Sandy and greaser Danny fell in love over the summer. After the summer holiday, they find out that they're now in the same high school, which causes conflicts and heartache for different people.

The Virgin Suicides

A group of male friends become obsessed with a group of beautiful sisters who are sheltered by their strict, religious parents after one of them commits suicide, but the sheltering ends up in more tragedy.

Romeo & Juliet

Shakespeare's famous play about two teenagers from rivaling families who meet, fall in love, and fight for their love despite their parents being enemies. There are different filmed versions of the tragedy.

Dead Poets' Society

Students at a boarding school meet Professor Keating, their new English teacher, who tells them of the Dead Poets Society, and encourages them to go against the status quo. Each, in his own way, does this, and is changed for life.

American Beauty

Parents and their children living under the same roof but having completely different lives. Daughter Jane is embarrassed about her parents while developing a happy friendship with a shy boy next door named Ricky who lives with a dominating father.

Forest Gump

Forrest Gump has both psychological and physical challenges in his young life, and he grows up experiencing the changes of the 1950s, 1960s, and 1970s, ending up accomplishing great things, including falling in love with a girl who does not feel the same way about him.

Donnie Darko

Teenager Donnie Darko tries to deal with people in his town, like the school bully, his conservative health teacher, and a self-help guru, while hearing the voice of an imaginary six-foot-tall bunny.

BE AWARE OF LIFE PHASES

How we look and the age we signal are important to many people. But looks are not the only key to well-being and feeling good about oneself. How we feel about our different life phases is equally important. This is why it is important to learn how to adjust to a new life phase.

Turning forty, fifty, or sixty years old represents not only biological changes, but also psychological changes. We may become aware that other people react to us in new ways, and we ourselves may observe changes in how we think and what is important to us. This is part of a natural process that most people experience. Of course, we may not be happy about it, and it can cause stress and depressive thoughts.

Growing older gives many people more insight into themselves, and some people become more confident and sure of themselves with age. But growing older also represents a loss or can be viewed as a loss—of youth, of good times, of health. We may not like it, but if we know how to say a proper "good bye" to the life phase that is over, we are likely to feel better about our next life phase. A proper good bye is quiet and invisible, and may take some time, maybe a couple of years or more.

People who are in denial of the changing life phases often get mental health problems because they do not acknowledge their loss, and thus they avoid the feelings associated with what they have lost.

Loss may be a dramatic word to use in this respect, but loss reflects that to some people it can be dramatic to turn fifty, sixty, or seventy and retire from the workplace and realize that there are fewer chances to do what you want to do in life.

Using the word loss also indicates that there can be a need for a grieving process when all these changes happen. Grieving is an unpleasant feeling, but when handled as a process of change, it can lead to new insights, new life skills, and a new outlook on life.

The more literally you can say good bye to what you have lost, the better chance you'll have of getting through the entire grieving process without mental health problems. This may involve stating one's loss to oneself, either by verbalizing it or writing about it. Sharing these thoughts with people who are or have been in the same situation can be beneficial—if they have adjusted well to their new life phase.

Grieving takes time. It may take weeks or months, but verbalizing the loss one is feeling to oneself and to close family and friends are the most important steps you can take to move on with your feelings.

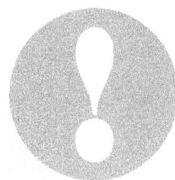

On your way to looking younger

❖ How old you look is also influenced by your thinking.

❖ Stay tuned in to what goes on among people younger than yourself.

❖ Let music, books, and movies be an inspiration to stay youthful.

Getting Started

CHAPTER FOCUS
❖ Golden rules
❖ Planning
❖ People's comments

Now that you have an overview of how to look the age you feel rather than your biological age, it is time to get started on looking younger. You have to decide what will work best for you, and what you feel comfortable doing. Do you want to make just a few adjustments—or do you want a complete makeover? No matter what you decide, here is some helpful insight that will help get you started.

On television and in magazines, we can watch or read about people getting makeovers. Not all of these makeovers are about looking younger; many are about "dressing right" or dressing in a certain style. But there is no doubt that the makeovers that give the most striking results are the ones that do the most visually in the shortest time.

Now it is *your* turn to get a makeover! The best way of being successful at looking younger and getting the most striking results is also by following all the advice presented in this book in a relatively short time, say, a couple of months. It is probably only then you will get *Wow!* responses.

There may be several reasons why it may take longer than a couple of months, though. It costs money to buy new clothing, and you do not get a fitter body or lose weight in a short time. Also, maybe you do not feel the need to take all options mentioned in this book into account. You may choose to just use some of the information right now. At other times, you may want to use other parts.

If you are in doubt how to begin to look younger, start with Chapter 10 about facial hair.

But before starting on looking younger, let's have a look at what are NOT age revealers. Each of us has a beauty ideal, and in society, there are always certain prevalent beauty ideals. They will change from time to time, but they are visible everywhere we look. Looking younger in this book is not just about a certain beauty ideal. There are many elements in a person's appearance that have nothing to do with looking younger but are about a certain beauty ideal or about looking sexy.

What Are Not Age Revealers

The following elements in a person's appearance have nothing to do with looking younger. You have not found information on these issues in this book simply because they have no influence on looking younger. They are visual signals that are neutral age revealers. Having a gap between your teeth does not say anything about your age.

- ☑ Being pale
- ☑ Buttocks size
- ☑ Chin shape
- ☑ Ear size
- ☑ Eye color
- ☑ Feet size
- ☑ Gap between teeth
- ☑ Hair color
- ☑ Lip size
- ☑ Moles
- ☑ Nose size and shape
- ☑ Scars
- ☑ Skin problems

Many things about looks and beauty are not actually about age. If you are not happy about your appearance, this may affect how you approach life. Then you have to find out if you want to do something about what bothers you, what can be done, and plan what you want to do about it. Changing this will not automatically make you look younger, but you may end up looking more beautiful according to your own—and other peoples'—beauty ideals. It is important to be aware that you can look younger without changing what bothers you from a purely visual point of view because many of the things that may bother you could be age neutral.

This book presents many ways to look younger, but if we get to the core of it, there are Ten Golden Rules about looking younger. If you start by paying attention to these golden rules, you have a very good starting point.

The 10 Golden Rules of Looking Younger

The slimmer you are, the younger you look.

The fitter you are, the younger you look.

The more fashionably you dress, the younger you look.

The more fashionable accessories you wear, the younger you look.

The fewer wrinkles you have, the younger you look.

The whiter teeth you have, the younger you look.

The more hair you have, the younger you look.

The less gray hair you have, the younger you look.

The less body hair you have, the younger you look.

The more groomed facial hair you have, the younger you look.

Because not everything may be relevant, you need to make your own individual plan. You can do so by using this Easy-planner Checklist.

Easy-planner Checklist
1. First find out what you want to do.
2. Decide when you want to do it.
3. Do it.
4. Did it achieve what you expected?

Often, it will become more real if you write down what you want to do.

What I Want to Do	When I Want to Do It	Done or Not Done	How It Made Me Look and Feel

Your own comfort about the changes is the most important thing. Of course, it is always nice to get positive responses from other people. Some will volunteer their comments, but you have to prepare yourself that they may not always be positive. That does not mean that you have not achieved what *you* wanted and what this book is about. Actually, you may have achieved it too well. Some people do not like changes (even in other people), some will be envious of you because you look younger, some will feel that your efforts are unnecessary, or that you look ridiculous. There may be dozens of other explanations for negative comments. In order to find out how you should react to negative comments, try first to figure out the person's motive for saying what he or she does. While envy is unpleasant when we are confronted with it, it is a fact of life. When we are confronted with it, one way of dealing with it is accepting it as the other person's problem.

If you want to find out if you have succeeded in looking younger, ask people whom you trust to tell you their perceptions of you. This can be people that you already know—or it could be people that you have never met before or just barely know. When you start getting the same comments again and again, you are probably getting answers you can trust.

If you get comments that you can use, it is a good idea to keep track of them, especially if they make you feel good; they are worth remembering. You can use this log to keep track of comments.

Comments on My Look

Name	Comment	My Comments

Name	Comment	My Comments

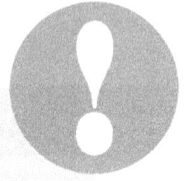

On your way to looking younger

❖ Not everything in this book will work for you—
   focus on what will.

❖ Looking younger is not about adapting to all or
   certain beauty ideals—only the ones that make
   you look younger.

❖ Be prepared for both positive and negative
   comments about your youthful look.

❖ Consult the tools and guidelines in this book from
   time to time to see if something new has become
   relevant to you.

About the Author

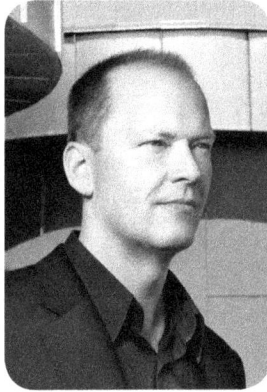

Henrik Vejlgaard, M.Sc., M.A., is the author three books: *Anatomy of a Trend*, *The Lifestyle Puzzle*, and *Style Eruptions*. The books document how changes in style and taste take place, and how we communicate with the clothes we wear.

He coined the term "age-elasticity" in the late 1990s and became an expert in understanding the new concept of age, i.e., that there is a huge difference between biological age and self-perceived age.

He is also the author of *Look Younger Without Surgery*, the women's version of *Look the Age You Feel*.

Other Books by
Henrik Vejlgaard

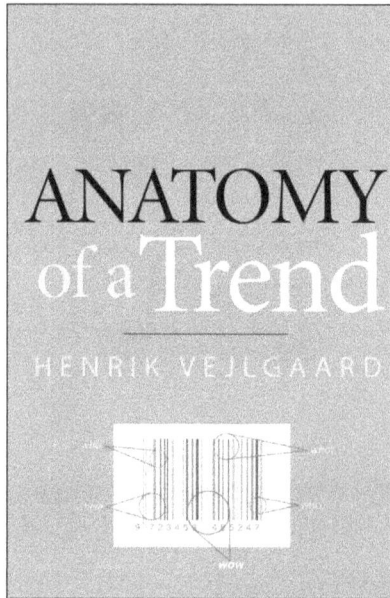

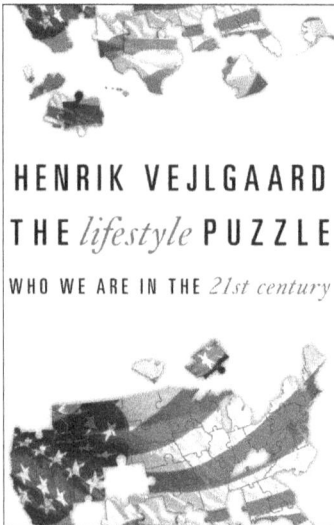

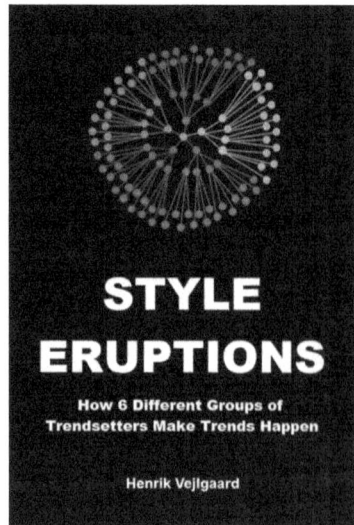

ANATOMY
of a Trend
HENRIK VEJLGAARD

HENRIK VEJLGAARD
THE *lifestyle* PUZZLE
WHO WE ARE IN THE *21st century*

STYLE
ERUPTIONS
How 6 Different Groups of
Trendsetters Make Trends Happen

Henrik Vejlgaard

www.ingramcontent.com/pod-product-compliance
Lightning Source LLC
Chambersburg PA
CBHW031208270326
41931CB00006B/466

9 7 8 1 9 3 9 2 3 5 3 6 7